Royal K. Kile
Humanitarian
Betrayed and Persecuted

All rights reserved. No part of this publication may be used, reproduced, transmitted in any form or by any means, electronic, mechanical, photocopying, recording or otherwise stored in a retrieval system, without the prior written consent of the publisher. To do so is infringement of the copyright law.

By
Gerald F. Foye

R.T. Plasma Publishing
9857 Old Ridge Road
Spring Valley, California
91977-3462
USA

Copyright January, 2001
First printing March 2001
Revised second printing March 2002

ISBN 0-9659613-3-8

CONTENTS

	Page
Dedication	2
Disclaimer	3
Caution	4
Introduction	6
Electronic energy devices	8

Chapter

		Page
1	John Crane (Rife Revival)	9
2	John Crane (Muddied waters)	19
3	Rife - Hoyland (Beam Rays Affair)	25
4	Fictional Story	29
5	Royal Raymond Rife	33
6	Unacceptance	45
7	An Intriguing Individual	51
8	Modern Medical Marvels	69
9	Fishbein, 'The Great!'	73
10	Case History	77
11	Medical Testimonials	91
12	Doctor And Patient	95
13	Memoirs	101
14	Medical/Political Persecution	107
15	Miscellaneous Data	113
16	Mamie Ah Quin Rife	123
17	Frequencies and Theories	127
18	Construction Basics	135
19	Backtracking	141
20	Mysteries and Oddities	145
	Final Chapter — John Crane	147
	Strange Event	149
	Update	150
	Conclusion	151
	Serious Experimenters	153
	Resources	155

Dedicated to........:

The memory of Royal Raymond Rife, his unselfish dedication, his lifetime of endless hours of research and development, his contribution to mankind, all suppressed and in vain!

Royal Raymond Rife, man betrayed, persecuted and destroyed by the very people he thought he was helping!

And, to those who are dedicated to restoring the name and principles of the late Royal Raymond Rife into the pages of medical science.

To the historians who are slowly locating and fitting together critical pieces of the Rife puzzle.

To the technicians who are working silently in the background attempting to reproduce the microscope and the frequency emission method Rife used to kill disease causing pathogens.

To the supporters of Rife technology and all other forms of alternative healing methods in the constant battle against medical tyranny and hypocrisy!

Though it is tempting to offer acknowledgment to those diligent persons who have made important contributions by listing names, to do so might bring the wrath of the 'system' down on them! Suffice it to offer silent tribute!

Disclaimer

The author is not building or selling Rife type devices or treating people with such devices. The purpose is not intended to market alternative treatments, products, remedies, equipment or devices.

None of this information is to be used in lieu of proper conventional medical treatment, diagnosis or other conventional medical services.

The material content is for reading and evaluation of the history of Rife and related technology. Going beyond reading and attempting actual application will place that person in the category of experimentation. Any form of experimentation may be hazardous.

Frequency treatments may possibly be dangerous. It may be possible frequency treatment could cause an expansion of tumor growth under incorrect conditions.

If a person has any doubts, fears, prejudices or any concerns over the use of such treatment or devices; they should not proceed beyond reading the material.

An experimenter must accept full responsibility for possible failure and subsequent harm to themselves or others.

There is no intent to imply frequency emission devices will cure anything. Any claims to 'resolve' health issues apply only to the author's specific, personal applications (which include unsubstantiated personal opinion); and, does not offer scientific evidence, or proof of cure, since that would require rigorous testing, including the test of repeatability, which has not been performed.

Caution:

A word of caution is in order for anyone who might attempt to apply this technology!

Information in this publication is based on research of historical documentation, news articles, court records, internet data, library records, and other sources relating to Rife plasma emission resonant frequency technology. The author has done his best to be factual, to the point, in non-technical format. The one fictional, 'moralized' chapter is designed to interest the reader in further investigation of their own.

The author has personally experimented with Rife plasma frequency emission technology! Some results were astounding — instant, without side effects. The author is convinced such technology offers great potential, is safe and should be investigated further!

The author is not a medical practitioner nor researcher, not an electronics technician and in no way profits from Rife technology devices or treatments.

The author has found the technology to be safe when administered properly although some minor negative effects might occur under certain circumstances.

In addition, 'what works for one person, may not work for another'; or, 'what may be harmless for one person may not be harmless for another'!

Any form of research and experimentation is subject to failure and possible harm. Therefore, the researcher must accept risk and responsibility. Regulations by the AMA/FDA were placed in effect long ago to discourage unwanted concepts. According to the FDA, 'unproved' is synonymous with 'illegal'. FCC regulations must also be considered. Efficacy of Rife technology has been established, proven and documented as far back as 1928 and many times after. Yet, the technology has been placed on 'hold' and declared 'unproven' by the FDA. This is understandable considering the threat to the economics of the existing medical system; the billions of dollars it leaches out of our economy on an annual basis.

Medical research into acceptable and viable alternatives will be held back until the medical industry becomes civilized and truly practices the Hippocratic oath. Meanwhile, the Great Gods Of Medicine have determined it to be in the best interest of humanity to suppress radical concepts and continue to administer their brand of healing: drugs, surgery, radiation!

There are people who have discovered answers to many of our questions. People who have constructed electronic devices that work as well or better. But, they dare not pass on this valuable information in fear of receiving the wrath of the medical system, as has taken place so many times through the decades.

Alternative medical concepts are under constant scrutiny by medical watch groups. Alternative practitioners have been hounded, intimidated, jailed. Websites have been shut down.

For decades, many dedicated practitioners of viable alternatives have chosen to leave the country and practice elsewhere. Even then, the long arm of greed reaches out after them.

Legislation has been placed in motion to allow pharmaceutical giants to gain international control over all supplements, vitamins, herbal and alternative products and treatments.

The reader is encouraged to verify subject matter in this book by searching the library and internet. Key words: 'Codex', 'global harmonization', 'Rife technology'.

Introduction

This documentation is about Royal Raymond Rife and his sensational device for 'devitalizing' cancer and other major diseases. It explains the method, how it was developed, how it was proven to be effective and why is it not presently available? It also touches lightly on the never ending struggle between conventional and alternative medicine that so seriously affects our lives.

People who prefer the conventional medical system to dictate the terms of their health to them should follow that path. Doctors of conventional medical practices who prefer to follow the same narrow path and the dictates of their colleagues, have every right to do so.

But, there should be equality for those who prefer alternatives. The choice of health procedures and treatment should be up to each individual, should they chose to make their own decisions.

But, such is not the case. Liberal medical practitioners who step off the path, even slightly, are admonished and forced back in line. If they should attempt to ignore their peers, there is no limit the system will take to meter out their form of justice. Scores of medical practitioners have suffered the wrath of the medical system. The noose is always waving in the breeze, awaiting it's next victim. The general public naturally assumes anyone who is imprisoned over the issue of health procedures must deserve it. But, if they were to do their homework they might find a different story. A story of hostility and intrigue equal to the best of fiction.

All forms of alternatives are placed on the 'quackery' list and labeled 'unproven', (i.e. illegal)! It is ironic that, in other countries, where freedom is suppressed and abuses against humanity prevail, our representatives step in, confront issues and send troops if necessary. Yet, in the United States, similar atrocities are strangely ignored by the same representatives. Worse yet, the American public is apathetic. We should reflect on the warning of Abraham Lincoln when he suggested our nation can only be destroyed from within. Chilling words, when you consider them carefully.

The intent is not to speak against orthodox medicine; but, to point out that proponents of alternative medicine should be allowed equal rights. Let the public determine which route they prefer.

When one studies the history and background of such a man as Royal Rife and learns of the ordeals he suffered and the consequences of being a dedicated humanitarian, it becomes a traumatic and saddening experience. His life (as well as the lives of many of his followers) was destroyed by the very people he thought he was helping!

How can anyone deny the man his due place in history after such diligent efforts and marvelous discoveries? Was Rife simply a man in the wrong place at the wrong time? Or, is a more sinister force involved?

Monopoly is a formidable word. There can be no greater monopoly than one that uses government agencies and tax payer money, to forcibly administer its agenda.

Electronic 'Energy' Devices:

Numerous electronic 'energy' devices are labeled Rife devices, which may not be accurate.

A true Rife device is a ***radiant plasma resonant frequency emission*** device. A gas filled plasma tube serves as an antenna. Frequencies are radiated through the air within a given range (field). The field is roughly within 15 feet of the plasma tube. No wires are attached to the target. Technically, many targets can be treated at the same time, within that field.

Devices may contain one or more fields: E-electrical; M-magnetic; RF-radio frequency, light field (photon energy).

Pad devices are basic E-field frequency generators attached to the target via wires and electrodes.

Another variation utilizes electromagnetic energy (M-field) as a carrier for frequency waves by way of a hand held plasma tube extended with a wire connected to the source. This allows treatment of the target with direct application of the plasma tube.

One important feature of a frequency emission device is to permit the user to select specific frequencies 'within the range of the instrument'. Some devices do not allow frequency options. This places a true researcher at a disadvantage.

The author considers plasma tube devices to be most beneficial! Besides greater penetration, there seems to be unknown or unidentified beneficial components within the plasma emission that pad devices do not offer.

For the do-it-yourself type, computer programs are available allowing frequency selection, sequencing, specific pulse rates, duration settings and more.

It is important to select a unit to meet the users goal and comparing dollar value is very important.

Chapter One

John Crane (Rife Revival)

John Francis Crane, convicted and sentenced to Chino, California State Prison, April, 1961. John Crane, John Marsh and Lallas Bateson were charged with attempted grand theft, conspiracy to commit grand theft, and conspiracy to violate section 2141 of the business and professions code, the section prohibiting the practice of medicine without a license. They were convicted of all three offenses.

John Crane, born September 11, 1915, Elsinore, California. His mother died in 1950. His father was an engineer with the City of Elsinore.

Background: a practical, hard working man with a desire for practical education. Worked as a truck driver, coal miner, machinist, engineer and many, various jobs.

Schooling: Oceanside College, Riverside College, University of Southern California, University California Los Angeles, Aero Industrial Technical Institute, Lockheed-Burbank Trade School (all in California), plus a University in Alaska.

John studied: zoology, physics, mathematics, electronics, machine and tool design, operations, production and industrial engineering, surveying and related fields.

It appeared John had a goal and selected specific classes since his stay was often one half to one year of education at any one facility, other than the Lockheed Trade School where he went through a five year program in machine and tool. (*May also have been economics!*)

John stated that he could work in a number of fields such as, accounting, photography, sheet metal, machine and tool, and welding!

Miscellaneous information indicates John Crane had a sister. No further mention is made of his sister. John married while attending a University in Alaska. He divorced his wife in 1946. There were no children. He remarried in 1947. That union resulted in two children. John served in the military, 1945 — 1946, from which he was honorably discharged. John died, 06/06/95.

Going back to the early days of John Crane it becomes obvious John was a hard working man; and, of strong character and strong convictions. A review of the court proceedings indicate that John was extremely adamant in his determination to continue constructing his Rife type frequency healing devices and to continue spreading word of their benefits. He stood up against the court. He could have easily backed down, repented and avoided prison. But, that was not the way John did things. He even stated that he would consider leaving the country in order to set up operations elsewhere so Rife technology could be passed on to the benefit and future of mankind. Is this truly the character of a swindler?

Crane had met Rife and discovered the work and theories of Rife about 1950. Crane soon became enamored with the potential. Crane likely considered the financial prospects; although, it appears he had a genuine interest in the healing capabilities of Rife technology!

Initially, Crane constructed plasma tube devices based on the concepts of Rife as available to Crane at that time. The devices were cumbersome, costly, and definitely, not portable. A large bulky cabinet with internal and external components. The operator's panel consisted of large, cumbersome dials, of the era. A large phanotron tube (bulb) was mounted above, suspended from a support bracket. Overall height appeared to be about 4 - 5 feet. It was a complex and costly system. (*The above is based on a promotional film the author viewed.*)

Later, John created smaller, compact units. These units used hand held pads (contacts) instead of plasma tubes. Frequencies were directed by physical contact with the body. These were pad or contact devices. Crane contact devices were off-the-shelf frequency generating units, modified to generate square waves. These units did not use plasma tubes. This is where the so-called Rife pad devices appear to have entered the scene! However, the devices were effective!

Unfortunately, the name Rife was, and still is, applied to just about any and all electronic frequency healing devices of all shapes, forms and descriptions relating to health. Little of it is true Rife technology. And, as is true of so many other aspects of our modern world, charlatans have stepped in, abused and misused so-called Rife technology for profit. As in the past, it is still classified as 'quackery', even though Rife proved over-and-over, that his concept was viable and that it did work as he claimed.

Records indicate some of Crane's devices were placed in the hands of qualified medical practitioners for experimental use who were achieving promising results. So much so, that some of them were pushing for serious research of the units in hopes of receiving FDA approval. This brought word of the revival of frequency healing technology to higher medical authority. John Crane's marvelous devices had aroused the wrath of powerful influences! That nasty Rife concept had not been totally destroyed after all! **(Keep in mind, this revival was some twenty years after the initial suppression of Rife's work!)**

In order to market the units, John started a company called Rife Virus Microscope Institute. (Or, Microscopical Institute, depending on which files are read.)

John Crane knew it was illegal to treat people with his 'unproven' devices. He also knew he could not legally sell the units. But, the only way to prove the point was to get the units in the hands of needy people and prove the efficacy through actual application. John was also encouraged by reports from medical doctors of the efficacy of his devices. John, and associates, figured they could skirt the legal issues by loaning the units and receiving 'donations' to cover cost. The arrangement started off well; but, alas, word had gotten to higher authority that *someone out there was actually curing people who were advised by proper medical authority that they were supposed to be terminal.* Unknown to John Crane, a devious plan was set in motion.

The Rife Virus Microscope Institute was contacted by a lady who had heard reports of the Crane device and wished to procure such a unit. Unknown to John Crane, the lady had been appointed by the FDA to entrap John and his associates.

The home, and apparent headquarters, of Rife Virus Microscope Institute was raided, without a search warrant, so claimed John Crane. All records, products, equipment were seized. Sadly, this also included research data, magnetic tapes, equipment and devices that had, at one time, belonged to Royal Rife. According to court records, John Crane had purchased "all equipment from Royal Rife for $10.00". Possibly this was a result of Rife being subdued by alcohol and years of merciless pummeling by the FDA, AMA, Morris Fishbein and other infamous 'defenders of humanity'.

In court, John defended his actions. Fifteen witnesses were brought in who testified the units had helped their medical problems. *However, the court determined, "these people had not fully realized they had been victimized".*

John was admonished for his lack of patience in 'allowing time' for the units to be properly reviewed for medical approval. Although this line of thought may seem reasonable, how could anyone with limited finances be in a position to spend 10 - 15 years of their life, along with the required millions of dollars, to have their product properly endorsed? This is especially true when prejudice may be involved!

The three defendants were found guilty of the charges brought against them!

John Crane and John Marsh were unrepentant. The pair were convicted and sent to prison for a ten year term. John Crane was released in less than four years.

Lallas Bateson was firm in her convictions. After all, she had suffered a serious medical problem which would require removal of her colon followed by the ever present colon bag. But, she corrected her problem with Crane's device, did not require surgery and was sold on the merits of frequency healing. That is how she had initially come in contact with Rife Virus Microscope Institute. It is why she joined forces with the institute and held esteem and enthusiasm for her involvement. However, to avoid imprisonment, she agreed to 'repentance' and was given a ten year probation. She left the state shortly after.

Royal Rife had been called as a witness but did not show up as demanded. Rife had been previously and properly destroyed by the upper echelon of medical hierarchy and was in seclusion across the border. A deposition was taken but arrived too late for the trial.

One might speculate on this issue: Rife may not have wanted to cross the border for fear of being arrested. (*See reference to a similar event in the case history of renowned Dr. William F. Koch who was arrested after being deceitfully enticed back into the United States by his unscrupulous colleagues.*) Some also speculate that Rife's deposition may not have been favorable to John Crane for certain reasons. It is also obvious that many of the questions to be asked on the deposition were questions Rife may have preferred not to answer. Many questions appeared irrelevant to the court case but might well be 'extremely relevant to outsiders' who might possess the finances and influence to either utilize future development of Rife technology for themselves; or, control the patents with which they could prevent development. Once in court records, this valuable information could be openly accessed by anyone.

A review of the proceedings indicate many judgmental errors and prejudice. An appeal was made but denied. A request was made for return of all confiscated items but there is no record that any of it was returned.

There are notations in court records that the seizure of records denied the defendants access to vital evidence that would have supported their defense and that data and witnesses to the defense was ignored or refused as evidence by the court. But, according to a court review, none of it would have made a difference.

Court records as follows: "On the evening of November 17, 1960, affiant was at his home, at (xxxx), San Diego, California, when Willis A. Worley (who is a Senior Food and Drug Inspector for the Department of Public Health of the State of California) arrived with one Mary Alice Plain (who was in the employ of, or working in co-operation with said Willis A. Worley).

They secured entrance to my home by representing to me that they were interested in obtaining the use of a certain machine and training in its use, said Willis A. Worley representing that his occupation was that of a truck driver and said Mary Alice Plain representing that she was a housewife. After some discussion of the use of said machine, both of said persons expressed a desire to secure the use thereof and training in the use of it, and entered into negotiations therefore, after affiant had informed them that such machines were not for sale. Said Willis A. Worley then produced a warrant of arrest and stated that affiant was under arrest under said warrant. Thereupon Charles M. Duggie, a Food and Drug Inspector for the State of California, and two other men (one of them a member of the police force of the City of San Diego, and the other a photographer, both of whom would not state their names) forced their way into affiants home, and — under the direction of said Willis A. Worley, Senior Food and Drug Inspector for the State of California — began forcibly seizing the various articles of personal property,...."

The report further states: "That at no time did said Willis A. Worley, Charles M. Duggie, Mary Alice Plain, said policeman, said photographer, or any of them, produce or even claim to have or be acting under a search warrant for the search of affiants home or the seizure of any article found therein."

(Author's note): It seems the issue here must have been *warrant for arrest* and *warrant for search and seizure.* This appears to be a technical issue; although, technical issues are often quite relevant.

To complete the story: As in the arrest of Crane and Marsh, Bateson's Crane device was removed from her home without a search warrant. Bateson stated, that if she had a million dollars, she would trade it for return of her instrument.

Lallas Bateson (11/05/22 — 06/03/97), born in Sherwood, North Dakota to Knute and Hilma Flem. Lallas was the youngest of five children. She moved to California in 1940 where she met and married Leo Bateson in 1942. The couple relocated to San Diego in 1944. They had two children. They divorced in 1959. Lallas later remarried. Lallas left California following the court battle.

John Earl Marsh was born June 24, 1913 in Dayton, Ohio. He was the third of four children born to John and Bessie Marsh. He attended the University of Cincinnati for four years. Marsh married in 1937, had three children. John Marsh died in 1986.

John Marsh, second vice president of Rife Virus Microscope Institute, was the third culprit in the sordid affair of attempting to heal the ill without a license. Marsh met Crane in 1953 while both worked at Convair Manufacturing in San Diego.

Marsh had gotten a plasma unit into the hands of a medical doctor in his home town of Dayton, Ohio. Marsh claimed that doctor had discovered many favorable results while using the *Rife ray device* but the clinical data was not allowed in court as evidence.

Marsh had connections with the Mormon Church in Utah and was able to interest the Church in experimenting with a *Rife ray device*. However, Marsh soon had difficulty as accusations were registered against him in reference to immoral advances to women he was treating. It also seems Marsh told people he was **'*from outer space and sent to earth on a mission*'**. For what ever reason that statement was made, it was unfavorable and discrediting!

Marsh had also left a *ray device* in Utah under the supervision of Dr. Edward Jeppson, MD. According to Marsh, favorable medical data that was achieved in clinical research that took place in Utah also was not allowed as evidence in court. Marsh also stated that Jeppson was later forbidden to use the instrument in further research. Per the statement of Marsh, "*Jeppson proved the instrument to be successful and not harmful to living tissue, nerves, bones, etc.*"

It was further recorded that the FDA wished to retain as many *ray devices* as they could in order to place them on public display as examples of quackery. This was property the FDA had illegally 'stolen', according to John Crane. The material removed was unquestionably worth many thousands of dollars and Rife's research material has value beyond any dollar amount. Plus, keeping this information under wraps could be of great benefit to certain factions.

Points of interest:
*RVMI built and placed 34 units in the hands of doctors and other interested persons.
*Crane insisted that Marsh and Bateson were responsible for distributing the units after he requested they stop doing so.
*About the time of Crane's trial, Crane attended the trial of a local medical doctor who, at the age of 79, had been arrested for using one of Crane's frequency instruments and giving patients (illegal) '*Koch injections*' for cancer treatment.
*Although there is no record of confiscated items being returned, they obviously were returned at a later date.
*Court records state, 'Rife sold all his equipment to Crane for $10.00'. This is not totally correct. Other individuals had also purchased certain items from Rife!

Special Notations:
*John Marsh was a Mormon. The issue of sexual harassment caused Marsh to be excommunicated. In addition, the church was compelled to distance itself from the frequency healing experimental program.

*Defending attorney, Bertrand L. Comparet, performed his defense in a compelling manner; but, a review of court proceedings makes one wonder if the court had predetermined opinions. Although close to 50 defense witnesses were available, only a few were called and their testimony was largely ignored. The jury was instructed that the only issue to be considered was *practicing medicine without a license.* Whether the frequency devices worked or whether illness had been cured, was to be ignored. Bert was licensed to practice in 1926. In addition to private practice, Bert served with the district attorney's office from 1942 - 1947, after which, he returned to private practice as well as teaching law. Bert retired in 1976, devoting time to a nondenominational religious organization which he established. Bert died 10/13/1983. There were no known survivors.

*Crane's various business names: Allied Industries, Life Labs, Rife Virus Microscope Institute, John F. Crane Corporation.
*Crane had written and distributed 'newsletters' which accosted the honor of the existing orthodox medical system. That information was unfavorable in his court trial.
*Crane material primarily from court documentation and letters. Some information intentionally omitted to avoid people and places from being visited by curiosity seekers.

Chapter Two

John Crane (Muddied Waters):

Proponents of true Rife technology say John Crane 'muddied the Rife waters'! John did indeed 'muddy the Rife waters'! But, the question is why? Was it simply to capitalize on Rife technology by constructing cheaply made, portable devices and distributing them like hardware store items? Or, was it lack of direction on the part of his mentor, Royal Rife? To sort things out we must backtrack to the origin of Rife technology: Royal Raymond Rife, himself.

Over a period of many years, beginning in the late 1920's, Royal Rife attempted, over-and-over, to gain acceptance of his famous microscope, his theories of 'virus devitalization' and his frequency healing technology. Thumbing through the pages of history relating to Royal Raymond Rife, we find he absolutely did verify that his devices did work but failed acceptance of his peers!

Rife successfully treated critically ill patients under the strict supervision of qualified medical doctors. But, what was the outcome? Rife's technology was quickly 'buried' by monopolistic powers. With such power and financial backing it becomes an easy matter of placing 'lobbyists' in strategic positions to pass laws to favor and protect an industry.

Rife eventually became totally demoralized, dejected and depressed. He was thoroughly destroyed by the power of the medical industry, by Morris Fishbein (AMA) and by many others who let him down.

By the time Crane met Rife, Rife had been heavily seduced by the influence of alcohol and had already spent time in a sanitarium!

Further, Rife had already been victimized by previous and dubious, business schemes which further diminished his enthusiasm and weakened his will to continue. Several business ventures had been established to produce and market Rife Ray devices; but, had faltered due to improper procedures, improper management, greed and infighting among partners and investors. This added to Rife's frustrations!

This would suggest Rife probably was not capable or willing to guide Crane to produce a true Rife plasma device. In addition, electronics had dramatically changed which may have created problems that Rife could not deal with. (Keep in mind Rife was in his early 60's at this point and it had been thirty years since he first developed his original frequency healing device!) Crane also stated that Rife would not divulge the correct frequencies. It may be that Rife was holding back critical details at this point.

Other problems centered around 'associates' deviating from Rife's designs, altering devices, making unapproved changes, not following guidelines and often producing and selling units without Rife's testing and approval. This included Rife Ray Tube devices, Crane's devices and the Rife Universal Microscopes.

In addition, changes in FCC regulations restricted the operational bands that could be used for the carrier waves needed to transmit frequencies. (The carrier wave frequency is a component required to transmit the audio frequencies that Rife is believed to have used for devitalizing microbes. This is like radio stations, each has its own transmission band or wave length.) In the early days, it was stated Rife's frequencies were known to project a distance of twelve miles. There is indication Rife may have used different carrier for waves for different pathogens!

It is difficult to imagine the research value of the items seized by the law that initially belonged to Royal Rife. The years of painstaking effort, research and discoveries of one of the greatest men to pass over this earth, removed by people totally unqualified to understand the importance of what they held in their hands. (Although it is certainly obvious higher authority realized the importance and seized the opportunity to suppress it.)

The motion to have the court return the seized property was denied. Although, there is no (formal) record of the material being returned, John Crane seems to have eventually retrieved the bulk of it!

Among the items seized: years of scientific research data of Royal Rife, about 200 copies of published reports of the work of Royal Rife, 16-rolls of recorded magnetic tapes. The latter being recordings of various persons concerned in the research and experimentation conducted by Royal Rife over a period of many years. Plus, numerous electronic components and many other pieces of equipment. This is a partial list.

It is known that Rife Universal Microscopes were extremely complex and so were Rife's Ray Tube Frequency devices. Rife's theories, his devices, his concepts, are all buried with him.

There was previous mention of Crane being in possession of several Rife microscopes and original style frequency instruments. It is not clear if these were among items seized nor disposition!

*John Crane served a little over three years before being released following an appeal.

Since Rife refused to appear in court, a deposition for the trial was taken in Tijuana, Mexico in the office of the Consulate General of the United States. The deposition appears to have arrived too late for the trial and was not applied.

The deposition questions are recorded in court trial transcripts. However, the answers did not appear and were received from a different source. Therefore, authenticity cannot be verified. However, it certainly fits with other available material!

Q: What is the basic theory upon which you sought to find a means of killing pathogenic organisms?
A: *The theory of coordinative resonance with frequencies which I proved would kill microorganisms by electron transfer and internal stresses of pathogenic cells owing to electromagnetic forces.*
Q: What kind of pathogenic organisms did you study in these experiments?
A: *Tetanus, typhoid, gonorrhea, syphilis, staphylococci, pneumonia, streptococci, tuberculosis, sarcoma, carcinoma, leprosy, polio, cholera, actinomycosis, glanders, bubonic plague, anthrax, influenza, herpes, cataracts, glaucoma, colitis, sinus, ulcers, and many other virus bacteria and fungi.*
Q: What pathogenic organisms did you study in virus form?
A: *Cancer virus, typhoid, tuberculosis virus, herpes virus, b-coli virus, poliomyelitis virus, and about 40 other viruses that have never been isolated before.*
Q: About how long a period of time did your work/study of these viruses and proof of their pathogenic character cover?
A: *15 years on virus only!* **(Author's note: this is in addition to other pathogenic organism studies!)**

Q: Did you find whether some bacteria were capable of releasing a form of virus?
A: *Yes. Virus are released from bacteria just as a chicken lays an egg.*
Q: How did you determine this?
A: *By virus observation and cell study and virus photographs which I made and one which John Crane made a film of cancer virus which has been copyrighted.*
Q: What are some of the bacteria which you found to be capable of releasing a form of virus?
A: *Bacillus coli, tuberculosis, typhoid, and many others.*
Q: What is necessary in order to make bacteria and viruses visible under the microscope?
A: *First there must be high enough power to enable the observer to see them and second they must be identified by a frequency of light which coordinates with the chemical constituents of the virus or filterable form in question. To my knowledge there is only one instrument today which will even show these virus and that is the Rife Prismatic Virus Microscope which I built for this work. The electron microscope is a useless device for this study because the virus are killed instantly and you don't know what form you are seeing them in and generally appear as round balls of dried up chemical particles.*

In answer to a question as to how long Rife had studied bacteriology, the answer was: *40 years.*

Rife described *de-activate* as a term to indicate a virus may not be destroyed but rather will no longer reproduce. The author suggests the term *devitalize* may be in the same context!

(Page filler tidbit):

SDUT: (San Diego Union Tribune)

SDUT 12/12/2000
Doctors ordered: read the drug label
Doctors ignoring safety warnings...

(Internet)
FDA critical of Red Cross Blood Handling

Los Angeles:
...court awards boy malpractice award after he was severely disabled by negligent anesthesiologist who continues to practice...

SDUT 1/24/2001
Drug maker to pay $14 million in inflated-price case...

Chapter Three

Rife - Hoyland (Beam Rays Affair)

The Hoyland affair took place in the late 1930's, another dubious venture Rife was forced to endure. According to court records, (filed January 28, 1938) Philip Hoyland took action against Beam Rays, Incorporated.

The business was initially Aero Reserve School, Western Division, about November, 1935. Later, the name was changed to United Polytechnical Institute, (June, 1937). United Polytechnical Institute was operating under a licensed contract with the principal company, Aero Reserve School, Incorporated in Virginia. The purpose was to establish and maintain a school to teach aeronautics and allied subjects for the practical knowledge of airship design, construction and maintenance. In May, 1938, the name was again changed — Beam Rays, Incorporated. This was for the purpose of manufacturing and marketing the Rife Ray Beam device.

Philip Hoyland was a business associate of Rife. According to a letter written by Rife, Philip Hoyland had *"assisted Rife in designing better frequency devices"*. This would indicate Hoyland's expertise was in electronics. Philip Hoyland also appears to have been a business partner in Beam Rays, Incorporated.

Beam Ray, Incorporated had an exclusive agreement to manufacture and distribute Rife Ray Beam units, worldwide. However, it appears Hoyland took it upon himself to assign exclusive rights to a British firm to also manufacture and distribute Rife Ray Beam units worldwide, (except in the United States). When the British firm discovered the infringement upon their agreement, they took legal action against Beam Ray.

Hoyland also initiated action against Beam Rays in an apparent attempt to either gain control by demanding controlling interest through stock shares; or, (as a business partner contemplated) to dissolve the corporation in order to gain complete control. The case then developed into a battle over stock control and thus corporate control.

(December 6, 1939), plaintiff was Philip Hoyland versus Beam Rays, Incorporated. Defendants and cross defendants were Beam Rays, Incorporated. Cross defendant, Philip Hoyland and Royal Raymond Rife.

From court records: ".., but, it is true that said strife and dissention is caused wholly by the acts and conduct of the plaintiff herein. That it is true that defendant corporation made a contract with certain British persons, sub-licensing them to make and distribute Rife Ray Machines within the British Empire and that the plaintiff was employed by defendant corporation as its technical adviser; ..."

The gist of the comments were that the plaintiff was to supply the British firm with all the plans and information so the British could manufacture Rife Ray Machines. But, that the plaintiff failed to supply the plans and information.

The end result was: "That cross-complainant, Beam Rays, Incorporated, is entitled to judgment against the cross-defendants Philip Hoyland, C.R. Hutchinson and Royal Rife, adjudging that the license granted by said cross-defendants to said cross-complainant to manufacture and distribute Rife Ray machines and to sub-license other persons to manufacture and/or distribute Rife Ray machines at any place in the world, and that when said license was reduced to writing by the inadvertence and mutual mistake of the cross-complainant and the cross-defendants, said written contract of license failed to state that it was exclusive, and cross-complainant is entitled to a judgment..."

"That plaintiff Philip Hoyland should take nothing by his said complaint, and that the defendants and each of them should have and recover of said Philip Hoyland their costs and disbursement therein incurred."

There was comment by Rife that ***Hoyland had shipped two frequency instruments to England, improperly wired, "in order to obtain a trip to England"***!

Before and during the court battle the British firm was continuously demanding correct frequencies (MOR's) for their research. They had a Rife (Beam Ray device) but it did not perform properly. The information was not sent. This was due to speculation on the part of Rife counterparts that the British firm was more concerned in obtaining the frequencies than the actual device. This was because they had an electronics engineer who claimed he knew more about frequencies than Rife and had himself constructed a frequency healing device that he felt was as good or better. All he seemed to need were the actual MOR's.

Once again Royal Raymond Rife was forced to become embroiled in an affair which he had nothing to do with — an attempt to wrest control of the device away from him. Rife had become an unwitting defendant. It is also noted Royal Rife did not appear on his behalf at the inquiry. *(Later, it was said, Hoyland admitted to an error in judgment! Some speculate Hoyland was unwittingly seduced by 'outside influences'!)*

During the trial Rife had made arrangements to go to England to straighten out the misunderstanding and to get his equipment properly working. He intended to do this for the benefit of the British firm as well as to clear his name and good intentions. Rife made the arrangements but failed to complete his goal as he was subpoenaed for the pending trial and was unable to leave.

When the trial was completed, Rife was able to re-establish negotiations with the British firm. In particular, Rife was on very hospitable terms with a Doctor Gonin of England who was a staunch supporter of Rife. Gonin did his best to establish Rife's frequency healing method in England. Rife and Gonin corresponded and maintained friendly contact with one another for several years until the death of Dr. Gonin.

The British negotiations continued until World War Two brought the affair to a halt.

*Correspondence, from England 1938: "The machines from the Beam Ray Company arrived only last Monday, and are completely useless as far as we are concerned. In many cases the wires were not even attached or soldered. Nor has Hoyland sent us the exact frequencies."

1939: "The wave form of the machine was full of harmonics. The machine we saw in San Diego was free of harmonics. For all I know, this may be important. Further, these machines were faulty in other ways, faulty connections, etc."

*Special notation: It was later stated by an associate of Rife's (Benjamin Cullen) that it was after the Beam Ray affair that Rife began 'drinking', which was to become such a destructive factor in Rife's life!

Chapter Four

Fictional Story

Americans love fiction, so let's set up a fictional presentation which we hope will be of interest and perhaps, a lesson to be learned. Let's go back to the old west with the good guys and the bad guys.

Roy, local cowboy and inventor, is in his barn working on his latest project. A fellow cowpoke rides in, "Roy, thar's an Easterner with fancy cloths and a fancy hat just got off the train. He's a lookin' fer ya!"

As the cowpoke rides off, Roy peers out the window and notes the mysterious stranger talking to a local, he seems to be asking directions. The local points the way and the stranger heads for Roy's barn.

There's a knock on the rustic door as Roy reaches for the latch. He opens the door. Without a greeting the stranger enters, carrying a large satchel. He walks over to Roy's work bench, clears an area and thrusts his satchel on the bench.

"You Roy, the inventor?", the stranger asks.
"Yes sir, I'm Roy! Who are you?"
"Name's Squid. I'm here to present you with an offer you won't be able to refuse!"
Roy takes a step back, he's puzzled!
"I don't get it. What kind of an offer are you talkin' about?"
"An offer for your new horseshoe design!"
Roy is set back a bit. He has to clear his brain and analyze the situation.
The stranger becomes more aggressive, he raises his voice.

"Roy, I represent the Association of Industrial Horseshoe Makers of this country!"

"So, what does that mean to me?", Roy asks!

"We heard about your new revolutionary horseshoe and we want to make a deal," states the stranger in a louder voice! "Got the papers here fer you to sign!"

Roy is pleased with the turn of events. At last, the world is coming to Roy's door. Roy considers he will finally get the recognition he deserves, a chance for the world to learn of his latest invention; and, of the many other important inventions he hoped to eventually introduce to the world. Things that will make life easier for the masses, a little profit for himself and a rightful place in the history books. Roy had worked hard to get this far, long days and nights, blood, sweat and tears.

"Well, it's about time!", Roy said to Squid. "What sort of deal do you have in mind?"

"Very simple! You turn over your invention to me, personally!"

Roy is startled: "And, what does it get me?"

"Simple," says Squid. "For nine years you get nothing. Then, after that, if we determine your horseshoe is all we hear it is; then, you get ten percent of the profits and later we might even give you more."

Roy is flabbergasted. He has to sit down and go over the events in his mind. There is a long silence before Roy speaks again.

"I've poured my heart and soul in my inventions. It's taken every nickel I have. Friends have helped or I wouldn't have gotten this far. I can't accept that. I don't understand what's going on!"

"Roy, you've got to understand the dilemma your invention is creating. Horse owners have used conventional horseshoes for decades. Your 'better horseshoe' jeopardizes an entire, nation wide industry. Your new horseshoe could put thousands of conventional horseshoe makers out of business; jobs and lives are in jeopardy. Horseshoe research laboratories would be shut down."

"Wait a minute", responded Roy as the impact settled in. "Other horseshoe makers have had greater opportunities than I for designing improved horseshoes; yet, they haven't. Where does all that time and research money go?"

"Roy, you don't get the point! They may have developed horseshoes better than yours but they can't afford to create a horseshoe that would put themselves out of business!"

By now, Roy was deeply upset, angry, confused! He could tolerate it no longer. He refused the absurd offer and firmly requested that Squid get back on the train and inform the horseshoe industry that Roy was not going to turn over his invention to anyone under such ridiculous circumstances!

As Squid headed back to the train depot, he shouted, "Roy, you made a mistake not accepting our offer. You and your better horseshoe are done, finished, buried!"

Roy was shaken by the ordeal. Until now, Roy had never seen the inside of the local saloon; but, this day was different. The swinging doors clattered behind as Roy headed for the bar.

Months later another stranger arrived in town. He too was interested in locating Roy.

The Sheriff questioned this new stranger, "What you want with Roy?"

"I got a warrant for Roy's arrest!", answered the stranger.

The Sheriff couldn't believe what he was hearing: "An arrest warrant for Roy? What ever did he do to deserve this?"

"Practic'n horseshoe mak'n without a license, that's what!", the stranger quickly replied.

"What? Git outta town, stranger, afore I lock you up", shouted the Sheriff in anger!

Shortly after the stranger departed a local cowpoke walked over to the saloon where he found Roy. "Roy, take a look at this!" He handed Roy a poster that he had just removed from the wall of the train depot. It was a 'wanted' poster with Roy's picture on it.

A few months later, another stranger arrived in town. "Anyone seen Roy?", he asked. There were blank stares from the locals. Finally one local responded: "Mister, if you want to see Roy you'd best head on over the border into Mexico, 'cause that's where he's a hidin' out now. He went across the border right after his barn mysteriously burned to the ground! But, don't ask us exactly where he is, 'cause we won't tell ya if we did know!"

*So, goes the saga of Roy and his 'better horseshoe'! Absurd? Perhaps! But, if one does their 'homework', they might tie the moral of this story in with harsh reality!

Chapter Five

Royal Raymond Rife

Royal Raymond Rife, also known simply as Roy, was born May 16, 1888, died August 5, 1971. He died virtually alone and penniless, 'according to The Daily Californian, dated Wednesday, August 11, 1971'. Another publication stated that Royal Rife died in his home at 5555 Grossmont Center Drive, La Mesa, California. His home? An interesting statement since that is the address of a very large hospital complex in the San Diego area.

His remains rest in Mount Hope Cemetery (San Diego, California) where a single tombstone with a double entry engraved upon it identifies both Raymond Royal Rife and his first wife, Mamie Ah Quin Rife. Mamie's inscription: October, 7, 1886 - October 8, 1957.

Rife's father, Royal Raymond Rife, Sr., was born in 1867, in Ohio. Rife's mother, Ida May Cheny Rife was born in Cresion, Iowa. Ida May and Royal Rife, Sr., were married about 1886 in Fontanelle, Iowa. Royal Raymond Rife, Jr., was born in Elkhorn, Nebraska. A sibling, prior to Rife, Jr., apparently died before Rife was born.

Royal Raymond Rife, Jr's venture into the world did not start off well as his mother, Ida May, died less than a year after he was born — early 1889. Royal Rife, Sr., unable to work at his trade as a mechanical engineer and care for his newly born son at the same time, turned Rife Jr., over to his aunt, Nina Culver Dryden who was about 19 years at the time. Nina came from Ottumwa, Kansas. Rife remained with Nina until 1905.

Rife appears to have relocated in San Diego in 1906. A few years later, in 1912, Rife married Mamie Ah Quin, a proud lady from a prominent, wealthy Chinese family! There is considerable history of the Ah Quin family located in the Chinese Historical Society in San Diego. Unfortunately, the Society has little information on Royal Rife. They are as curious about Rife as we are! However, it is obvious 'someone' honored both Raymond and Mamie with a very nice memorial headstone.

How did such a man, who was an obvious genius; and, who offered great hope for mankind, end up a penniless alcoholic?

Upon arrival in San Diego in 1906, Rife became chauffeur for industrialist and entrepreneur Henry Timken of Timken roller bearing and axle fame. Timken had a retirement home in San Diego as well as other extensive real estate holdings. Rife was quartered in a small apartment over the garage. Rife had a fascination for microscopes and related optics and loved to tinker. Rife promptly dedicated a corner of his quarters to his hobby. Rife's interest in optics soon caught the attention of Henry Timken who was quick to realize Rife's potential and allowed Rife to expand his capabilities by sending Rife to The Zeiss Works, in Germany, the world's leading optical industry, for further studies. Rife studied for 6 years under the leading technician, Hans Luchel (or, Luckel).

Back in his laboratory in Point Loma, the training Rife received, combined with Rife's own genius and creativity, sent Rife on a path of his own in the field of microscopy. Rife was not satisfied with existing technology of the era. In addition to inadequate magnification, only dead organisms could be viewed due to heat generated by lighting and necessity of chemically staining organisms in order to be viewable. Rife wished to study organisms in their live, natural state.

Rife spent years developing a series of complex microscopes in order to create the 'Universal Microscope'. The final scope weighed about 200 pounds and consisted of over 5,000 parts. The unique feature was the ability (for the first time) to view microorganisms in their live state. Instead of staining with chemicals, the organisms were stained with resonant light frequencies which caused them to become 'luminescent', viewable; and, without killing them.

The unique light staining method was the key to success. Specially made prisms were ground to extreme precision. The prisms were mounted in such a way that they could be rotated, and precisely adjusted, to tune the light frequency to that of the organism, causing the organism to become luminescent.

The Rife Universal Prismatic Virus Microscope, had magnification capabilities far greater than any scope of its time and, indeed, for decades after. The tremendous magnification, coupled with the light staining technique, opened an entirely new window into the secret world of organisms and viruses that had never before been seen.

One unfortunate aspect of Rife's amazing scope was extreme difficulty of operation coupled with the need of extraordinary patience and time consuming demands. Rife's dedication allowed him to gaze into the scope for hours on end as he explored this previously invisible realm. Other researchers lacked the skill and patience required to operate such a delicate and vulnerable instrument. Indeed, some researchers had such limited success that they suggested the scope to be useless.

Eventually, many technical articles were published in various scientific journals of the day expounding the merits of the scope and the new and exciting discoveries it unveiled.

With the power of the scope, Rife was able to isolate viruses that caused specific diseases. He was able to watch life cycles as one form transformed into another. This was termed pleomorphic. He was amazed to discover that minute particles, barely visible even under the extreme power of his scope, were in fact, viruses. He could eventually identify such organisms by color.

Organisms were proven to have an oscillatory rate; or, more simply, a specific and unique frequency, as proven by illuminating them with resonant light frequencies. This allowed Rife to expand his discoveries by working toward the cure of devastating disease.

By painstakingly determining a mortal oscillatory rate (MOR), and training that frequency on a given virus, Rife found the virus could easily and quickly be destroyed. This is selective in the respect a specific virus can be destroyed without harming surrounding tissue. The frequencies might cause the viruses to literally explode. (Much the same as the opera singer shattering a glass with a specific note — frequency!) Or, certain organisms would become immobile and, "jam up like logs". This process was termed 'devitilization'.

Rife went on to perform more complex issues by actually creating cancerous tumors (in rats) and then 'devitalizing' the tumors by this process. He was able to control cancer predictably and with 'repeatability'. (This is one of the issues fought then, and today over Rife's process — that is, repeatability.) Rife repeated critical experiments hundreds of times before he would document them in his record manual!

Rife went even further as he was able to prove that virus forms could be altered with chemicals. Thus, he could create disease producing viruses by manipulation of chemical structures. Again, he proved this over-and-over.

Research continued. More astounding discoveries were made. Rife's minority of supporters became more enthralled with these findings. Still, the announcements fell on the deaf ears of dogmatic, medical science.

It is uncertain how Rife discovered the ability to destroy microorganisms with frequencies. However, it would seem an integral part of his research. Since Rife utilized frequencies to illuminate viruses with his specially designed prisms in his Universal Microscope, it would be reasonable to assume the next logical step would be to use frequencies to resonate microorganisms to such a degree they would be destroyed, (devitalized).

Others suggest Rife used an Oscilloclast as his guidelines. The Oscilloclast was devised at an earlier date by Albert Abrams, who some claim to be the founder of frequency healing. The Oscilloclast is quite a different instrument. The Oscilloclast had already attracted the wrath of the existing medical establishment; thus, when Abrams later delved into radionics, he received even greater opposition and denouncement. Abrams built and distributed numerous Oscilloclast instruments throughout the country which were placed in the hands of medical practitioners of the era.

Whatever the case, Rife used frequencies to destroy disease causing microorganisms. To do that, Rife developed specialized equipment. This required painstaking research, especially to find the correct frequencies for the destruction of specific viruses or ailments.

Rife spent years at his research. He had to create equipment and methods of operation each step of the way. To prove his findings Rife developed a method to film what he viewed through his microscope. That alone was a considerable achievement for the era. Through it all Rife received little acclaim for his marvelous discoveries, his unending hours of research, his damaged eyesight.

Rife, and his supporters, some of them highly acclaimed and reputable medical doctors and medical researchers, proved over-and-over the efficacy of their findings. But, the years of dedicated, laborious work were in vain. Higher authority within the medical community had predetermined the world did not need Rife technology.

In the world of research and science, 'publishing' is an important criteria to gain a foothold in a competitive field — to become 'known'! Publishing in a scientific journal is an announcement of one's discoveries or hypothesis. Publishing may lead to glory, fame and fortune! On the other side, publishing may open the door to criticism, skepticism, ridicule, forcing the author into a defensive position. Not all who publish do it for credit. Some simply want others to follow through with what they have learned in hopes it may lead to something more beneficial. Rife was a humanitarian who faced the dilemma of a dedicated scientist who theorizes: "when money comes through the door, science flies out the window". Rife had little personal interest in fame and fortune, he was not interested in drawing attention to himself. He was generous, modest, unassuming. For these reasons Rife made a serious error which would prevent his wondrous works from being taken seriously — he failed to 'publish'! This proved to be a critical error on his part. (Publishing was mostly done by associates!)

Whenever Rife or his supporters attempted to gain acceptance or review of Rife's concepts and devices, they were met with scorn and contempt. The first issue would invariably be, 'show me his published works'! Even when it was suggested that skeptics visit Rife's well equipped laboratory to 'see for themselves', few would accept unless they saw the 'published works' first! Some would not accept what they saw, even after they saw it! Many declared what Rife had done as impossible; therefore, unacceptable. Dogma, protocol and higher education can sometimes 'close the mind' to new, radical or unfamiliar concepts!

Although most researchers consider publishing as a worthy goal and contribution to the field of science and research, Rife held quite a different view. In an interview Rife expressed the opinion that most authors of published research published "trash"! Rife felt the author's time would be better spent expanding their work and following through to a greater extent to further prove their work and apply it. He felt their 'papers' were often 'premature'!

Today, there are individuals and groups, working under difficult circumstances to reconstruct true Rife frequency healing devices. Some are doing it for profit, some are doing it simply to recreate a lost legacy and some are hoping to establish Rife's name in medical science — where it rightfully belongs.

It will be a difficult process as it is a matter of starting from the beginning since Rife's research data and devices, have been lost, stolen, hoarded or intentionally destroyed. Fortunately, some artifacts have been uncovered, like a few pieces of a large puzzle. Rife spent hours, days, months, painstakingly searching for frequencies for specific viruses. That information alone could save valuable time!

Many questions remain to create stumbling blocks. For example, what type of carrier wave was used? Did Rife purposely vary the carrier wave? Does RF play a role in the healing process or is it a side issue? What part do harmonics play in the process? What part do specific gases play in the output of the plasma tube? What about the use of multiple frequencies, electrical or magnetic fields? Did Rife really use audio frequencies? (Evidence indicates Rife did use audio frequencies; yet, some question that.)

The biggest question remains, why, after many decades, have Rife's theories and proof positive, been discarded and unaccepted? Why has further investigation been stymied? There are detractors who will state: "Rife's method does not work", even though they know nothing of the principles of the technology and have never seen or worked with such technology. Is it coincidence, lack of courage, lack of understanding? Is it 'protectionism' or something even more sinister?

*Note: In reference to Rife's discovery of killing organisms with generated frequencies, there is evidence that as far back as 1920 Rife was investigating the relationship of electrical treatment of diseases. He had discovered electrical characteristics and corresponding polarity of organisms.

By reviewing the works of Dr. Robert O. Becker the reader will discover an interesting parallel. In a more recent time period (decades after Rife's initial research) Dr. Becker investigated the involvement of electrical current, polarity and regeneration in living things. And, as Rife had already discovered, Dr. Becker found he also was rowing against the flow of dogmatic wisdom!

Even in modern times the medical system as a whole, has opposed the concept of electrical involvement of organisms and the issue of polarity!

*Over a period of many years Rife designed and constructed five 'specialized' microscopes. In addition, Rife designed, constructed or modified numerous other optical devices to meet research requirements.

*Rife began his work 1921—1922. Rife built his first microscope in 1922. He designed the Universal Prismatic Microscope which he constructed in 1933. Within a short time Rife had built four such microscopes, each with improved innovations.

*Rife designed a special microscope lamp in 1929 which he patented and sold. It was popular with many researchers engaged in microscopy.

Carl Zeiss (Optics):

A word about Carl Zeiss (1816 - 1888): Born in Germany, studied medicine. In 1846 Carl opened a shop in which he produced and repaired optical equipment for the University of Jena. Initially he specialized in the manufacture of microscopes. In 1886 he received the technical assistance of Ernst Karl Abbe, a mathematician and physicist, who later joined Zeiss as a business partner. The Zeiss facility developed a world renowned reputation for the manufacture of high quality optical equipment, particularly cameras and microscopes.
(Re: Microsoft Encarta 98 Encyclopedia.)

Timken Family:

Henry Timken, 1831 - 1909, must be given credit for his roll in sending Rife on a path to wondrous achievements. Henry Timken, a self-made entrepreneur, industrialist and inventor, held claim to 14 patents. Among them was the Timken Carriage Spring, which developed into spring and axle production; and later, the Timken Tapered Roller Bearing which truly set industry in motion. Prior bearings lacked durability, especially for heavy equipment and continuous use. Henry also invested heavily in realestate. Henry became a multimillionaire.

In 1887, Henry Timken had semi-retired in San Diego where he purchased a Victorian Mansion on the corner of First and Laurel. It was in San Diego where the association between Henry Timken and Royal Rife opened the way for Rife's genius. Henry saw great potential in Rife, encouraged Rife to follow his goals, and financed Rife to some degree.

Henry Timken had two sons, H. H. Timken and William R. Timken and daughter Amelia who married Dr. A.S. Bridges. The families successfully carried on with Henry's business ventures and land holdings.

In addition to business, fame and fortune, the Timken and Bridges families were nationally known for numerous and generous, philanthropic arrangements.

When Amelia died, February, 1940, her obituary mentioned Rife as a former employee. It also noted Amelia willed $50,000.00 to Rife to carry on his scientific research.

Although the Timken family financed much of Rife's work, Rife did hold claim to a number of patents of his own which provided financial support. One important patent pertained to a Timken related steel making process whereas Rife created a method of controlling and reducing defective steel which saved millions for the industry!

As an interesting side issue, it seems the Timken family owned a competition speedboat designed for International Speedboat Racing of the era. It seems Rife designed and headed boat construction which included German built engines. It is believed Rife piloted the boat to a speed record in 1915.

Rife Locations:
Rife worked in various places and facilities in the United States but his primary work was done in the San Diego area. John Crane also resided primarily in the San Diego area. Some locations used by Rife:
708 - 712 Electric Building, San Diego
Alcot St. (Lab)
Chatsworth Blvd
Zola Ave
The Chatsworth, Zola properties were likely part of the Timken holdings which were later sub-divided.

*Note: Street numbers have been intentionally left out to avoid present residents from being over run with curiosity seekers. Rife left nothing behind!
The Timken family held extensive property holdings. Rife lived in homes owned by the Timken family as well as utilizing Timken buildings as laboratories. During the second world war the large building, on Alcot, was leased for military (naval) research projects, some having to do with sound transmission in water and sonar experimentation. A group also operated out of this facility as part of the Bikini Atoll atomic bomb project. It has been reported (but unconfirmed) that Rife was a photographer on that project!

(Page filler tidbits)

SDUT 01/18/2001 (C1)
...Stock more than doubles on announcement of new drug...

...blood substitute trials boost stock...

Internet:
..mycoplasma experiments conducted in Texas prisons....

SDUT 9/21/2001
...Lawmakers plan to cut cost of prescription drugs...
(Is this the joke of the month?)

SDUT 11/24/1996
Auditors discover 4,660 hospitals repeatedly overcharged medicare...

Chapter Six

Unacceptance

There are people and powerful organizations still at work attempting to erase Royal Raymond Rife from the pages of science and medicine. At the same time, there are followers of Rife doing their best to revive and maintain Rife technology. But, guess which side has the most power, money and political influence?

What happened to the work of Rife, his inventions, discoveries, his proof? Why is the miraculous Rife technology being kept from us while we suffer the misery of horrible diseases. Did it really work as some claim?

Remember John Crane, the man who attempted to revive Rife technology in the 1950's and 1960's? The law entered his home, seized his personal property, records, equipment. Much of the equipment, records, tapes, film had been passed on to him by Royal Rife for the future of mankind.

This was not the only time intervention set in. In 1934, after an extremely successful medical research program was completed whereas '16 out of 16 terminally ill patients were treated and fully recovered using Rife technology', the results were quashed, records and equipment disappeared and the entire project swept under the carpet. The medical staff who witnessed the event and who honored Rife at a banquet, later, '*saw nothing and knew nothing*'. Some even went so far as to claim they had never even met Rife when, in fact, a photo of them gathered at the banquet was published in a medical journal with pictures and identification of the same individuals clearly in the photo.

Was the pressure of medical politics applied? Prominent medical doctors and medical researchers who had worked hand-in-hand with Rife, who had witnessed and assisted in documenting the research findings of Rife, who had viewed through his famous microscope, had seen the destruction of microbes by radiant technology, now declared they had never worked with Rife or his microscope or frequency devices. Even though some had placed their names on laboratory documentation acknowledging Rife research work, many later denied even knowing Rife.

They turned on Rife like a pack of wild animals. What a group of hypocritical, humanitarians! Could this be construed as conspiracy?

Rife was constantly forced to defend himself, his methods and his 'proof'. Fellow medical researchers, some prominent in their field, who dared to attempt to carry on Rife technology, were destroyed by their peers. Are these 'well meaning' people and organizations really out to protect the gullible public from the clutches of quacks and charlatans?

There is a lot at stake! For example, what would be the economics of a roomful of ill people being treated at one time, in a matter of minutes? What about the never ending 'business' of research and funding — research with little to show for the cost? What would happen to the numerous research facilities, such as universities, that rely on health care research funding? Why, after decades of research and heavy funding, has the cure for cancer not been found; or, for that matter, the common cold?

Regardless of ones belief in this matter, the public should be allowed a choice as to what method of healing they would prefer for their medical problem. Instead, we have an arrangement whereas health care terms are dictated to us along with the astronomical cost involved for which we have nothing to say. We are told, there are no options! The public is apathetic on this issue. Would our attitude be the same if our government forced us to attend a one world church?

'Unproven' is a nasty word, according to the FDA, which uses unproven as synonymous with illegal. Anyone daring to use 'unproven' methods, products, devices or procedures will suffer the wrath of the FDA, which includes licensed medical practitioners.

The interesting issue here is, a product or device may prove to be effective and harmless; yet, until it is approved by the FDA, it is still considered an unproven or illegal healing method. Does this make sense?

The cost of getting a product or device approved is an astronomical and time consuming arrangement for which a small independent company is not prepared. Does this arrangement support monopolistic concerns?

Over a course of several decades, Rife, and supporters, went through periods of trials and tribulation. Over-and-over, they proved the effectiveness of the Rife device. Many qualified experts were forced to perform experiments and treatments 'underground'. They worked and practiced in fear of their careers, reputations, and in some cases, their lives. Many qualified practitioners gave up in frustration as the result of peer pressure and intimidation. Careers were adversely affected!

Fortunately, some records relating to Rife, Crane and others, are still being gathered. The few papers, written by Royal Rife and often in association with qualified medical scientists, prove without doubt, the findings and effectiveness of Royal Rife's research. Such records clearly indicate that qualified medical supporters, in the past, did utilize the work of Rife, did utilize his method of frequency healing and did achieve desirable results. Best of all, the procedure is non invasive, without side effects and harmless to other bodily organs.

Many patients who found no relief through standard medical protocol found salvation using frequency healing devices. Many medical doctors worked with frequency healing devices, silently, in the back ground, building up evidence and case history files to support the efficacy of this wondrous healing method. There were failures; but, those failures were generally the result of having to deal with patients who had been discarded by orthodox medicine as hopeless cases, too far gone to receive benefit. Still, many of these 'hopeless' patients did survive after receiving frequency healing treatments.

Experiences such as this took place many times in the 50 or so years Rife attempted to introduce his wondrous technology to the world. The spirit of this incredible man was beaten and broken many times. The few followers that attempted to support Rife and encourage him onward were also eventually destroyed, including one 'mysterious' death. Rife tried desperately to pass unto mankind one of the greatest gifts of all! In the process, his own well-being was jeopardized, friends and associates turned against him. Is it no wonder Rife turned to alcohol to hide his anger, grief, humiliation?

An interesting paper, 'Proceedings Of The Staff Meetings Of The Mayo Clinic', July 13, 1932 offers fascinating insight into the efforts of Royal Rife and the highly qualified people with whom Rife worked.

***Many documents and bits of medical history are available to interested parties via the internet.**

The following is taken from correspondence written by Milbank Johnson to Royal Rife, December 19, 1935: "A meeting of the Special Medical Research Committee of the University of Southern California will be held Thursday, December 26........."
The names of several medical doctors are mentioned in the same correspondence. Ironically, many of these same doctors later denied having anything to do with the research program or Royal Rife.

Disappearing Records:
The above is in reference to the special clinical research trial where 16 patients were successfully treated using Rife's frequency healing method! The clinical study was arranged by Dr. Milbank Johnson and placed under the capable guidance of Dr. Rufus Von Klein Scmidt at the University Of Southern California, through a special medical research committee. The records of this historical, medical event conveniently disappeared. According to knowledgeable sources, Dr. (xxxx), a fellow researcher, carted off the records which ultimately disappeared. Dr. (xxxx) is the same doctor who later attempted to 'take over' Rife technology by constructing and marketing similar devices. Dr. (xxxx) seems to have gone so far as to use Rife's name on the building where the devices were being produced and marketed. Rife made the doctor remove the reference to his name!

*Rife did not approve of having his name attached to the frequency devices. He did not approve the name: Rife Device or Rife Frequency Device, or similar.

SDUT 1/25/2001
'Radiation reduces arterial re-blockage'...

From this article we learn: One to six months after heart angioplasty, 20 to 30 percent of the patients suffer re-blockage due to scarlike growth. But, according to a study, scarring after heart angioplasty can be reduced with radioactive beads inserted in the vessel wall after surgery. As with any procedure there are risks. **However, according to the study, the benefits outweigh the risks.**

It becomes more interesting when we learn the founder of the project received funding from companies making interventional radiation devices, holds patents and may receive royalties. In addition, an associate received grants from the company that made one of the FDA-licensed devices.

Chapter Seven

An Intriguing Individual

Let's take a look at the workings of the mind of Royal Raymond Rife. He was clearly a true genius with a variety of interests. Unfortunately, a lot of valuable information relating to Royal Rife has been misplaced, lost, stolen, destroyed, or hidden! Some is brief and incomplete. Piecing together a profile is difficult using only tiny segments of a large puzzle.

We know Rife had a fascination for microscopy which resulted in the subsequent development of the phenomenal Rife Universal Microscope. That alone required an unusually creative, inventive and demanding character.

The November 8, 1956 issue of a newsletter of the Instrument Society of America announced an event to be held at the Lafayette Hotel in San Diego at which the speaker was Royal R. Rife. The title, 'Optics In Industry and Medicine'. Text as follows: "Dr. Royal R. Rife has had over 50 years experience as a designer and builder of medical research instruments, including microscopes, spectroscopes, micromanipulators, stop-motion photomicrograph instruments, frequency instruments, optical tools and many others. **He is the co-inventor of the 'frequency instrument' recently approved by the public health service of the State of California for use in the devitalization of bacteria, virus, and fungi of all diseases and internal infections.**

Dr. Rife received an honorary PhD degree from the University of Heidelberg in 1913. He studied eye surgery for two years at John Hopkins University and did research work with Dr. A. I. Kendall, Dean of

Northwestern University Medical School and Director of Northwestern University Research Laboratory; and, with Dr. E. C. Rosenow, head of the department of Research Bacteriology at the Mayo Clinic, Rochester, Minnesota. He has published several papers in the medical field.

Dr. Rife holds 14 medals from the U.S. and foreign governments for special scientific work involving inclinometers, machine gun synchronization gears, variable pitch propellers and high altitude barometric scales.

Dr. Rife will discuss and illustrate the application, fabrication and design details of several types of industrial and medical optical instruments. His talk will also deal with the dimensional accuracy of lenses, prisms, and light beam systems. He will draw a comparison between the Universal Microscope and the Electron Microscope.

On display for their first public viewing will be one of the new 'frequency Instruments' and a 17,000 power optical microscope developed by Dr. Rife and his associates."

(Authors note: the author's copy of above is poor and some words may be incorrect.)

Let's review a couple points: Rife is mentioned as co-inventor and\or mentioned associates. That is an interesting issue. One thought is that sometime in the 1950's, Rife had sold all rights and equipment to John Crane for a few dollars! (Per Crane vs People court records.) Therefore, at this point Rife may have allocated himself as co-inventor and would also have to acknowledge his association with John Crane.

The 'new frequency device' was likely a product of John Crane's engineering and not one of Rife's true plasma frequency units. (This is speculation!)

It is of interest to note that as previously stated the California Department of Health had recently approved the frequency device. Yet, in the trial of Crane versus the People, the California State Department of Health appears to have denied they approved the frequency device.

Other Items of Interest:
*Rife was often referred to as commander or commodore. Although some speculate Rife may have served in the U.S. Navy, offering vague reference to naval intelligence, this remains an unconfirmed Rife enigma! However, laboratories at which Rife's presence was known did secret government work during World War II! Associates also believe Rife did secret government work in WW I.

*Designed and constructed his own aircraft and engines. (A letter indicates Rife was an expert in aeronautics; therefore, it is assumed Rife piloted aircraft.)

*An older publication (illegible date) refers to, "A scientific Sundial which not only tells the time anywhere on earth but also calculates longitudes and latitudes and determines the position of the sun and other celestial bodies, has been invented by two San Diego scientists, F.H. Ashlock and Royal Raymond Rife."

*The Tribune Sun, November 25, 1946: "...one of the most complete police laboratories in the land is taking form." The article continued by stating that it was being set up by Dr. Royal Rife who was also donating a valuable petrographic and polarizing microscope. It also noted that Dr. Rife was closing his laboratory in Point Loma. (Actually, Dr. Rife had started the forensic police lab several months prior — June, 1946.)

Rife was involved in a diversification of projects. Some were in conjunction with other companies such as Western Electronic Corporation of Los Angeles, California. This effort involved special optical lens Rife assisted in developing for M.G.M filming studio which offered greater clarification than lens available at that time. Another project of importance appears to have been a stereoptical lens of Rife's design. In addition, there was discussion of a zoom type lens Rife had designed which he used on one of his handmade guns. (Circa: 1937 - 38.)

As was often the case, Rife faced opposition from 'optical experts' who claimed the lens Rife had designed and constructed 'were impossible to achieve'. This seems to have been based on theoretical optical limitations that optical engineers could not resolve. (The same attitude and negative thinking prevailed over Rife's Universal Microscope!)

Correspondence, 1937: "I have talked over the possibilites of your lenses, especially the one we call the 'zoom' lens, (the one you have on your gun) with men who are recognized in the motion picture industry, and the answer is as usual, "There isn't any such thing", "it can't be done!"

Correspondence, 1938: "Dr. Jones has shown the photographs of the trees and the mountains in the background to several of the principles of M.G.M. and of course, they are all suspicious of trick photography. Witnessing the photographing would settle that."

Although Rife was supported and often funded by benevolent individuals, he was not totally dependent on such assistance. Rife was an innovator, inventor, craftsman and able to design and construct complex devices and equipment. He held patents on many such devices which supplied him with income.

Rife was a surgeon on the level we now refer to as microsurgery, as displayed by his famed, delicate surgery on his lab rats. As a result, his expertise (section cutting) was in demand by other researchers in the delicate preparation of slides to be used in microscopic research programs. For this type of microsurgery, Rife designed and constructed special equipment!

In addition, Rife developed The Rife Super Stethoscope and The Rife Bell Stethoscope which were in favor by numerous medical doctors. The Rife Super Stethoscope offered the advantage of use by two persons when desired (perhaps for training purposes) with greater sensitivity than other such devices. The Rife Bell Stethoscope offered the advantage of no sound distortion!

Also, Rife designed and marketed The Rife Microscope Lamp to meet the needs of low power as well as extremely high power applications.

He also held patents relating to processes and devices used in certain manufacturing facilities.

Rife designed, built and marketed many forms of optical devices: various microscopes, optical tools, microdissector, micromanipulator, spectroscopes, stop-motion photomicrograph, frequency instruments.

Although Rife (and later Crane and Rife) applied for grant funding for research, they were denied such funding!

Rife maintained a wide scope of interests: artistic, social, sports, humanitarian endeavors and a keen desire for scientific knowledge.

*Rife held **membership** in: Microscopical Society of Great Britain, American Society of Metals, Instrument Society of America. **Fellowship** in: Bio-Chemistry, (Institute for Scientific Research). **Honorary** degrees: Doctor of Philosophy, Heidelberg University; Doctor of Science, University of Southern California, 1935; **Honored** by Nobel Foundation, 5/6/1971.

*Rife **studied:** with optical technician Hans Luckel at Zeiss optical industry, in Germany; bacteriology at University of Heidelberg as well as John Hopkins University; (studied eye surgery two years).

*ABCResearch**: 1931, first announcement of cancer virus isolation; 1949, again announced isolation of cancer virus; by 1933, Rife had isolated over 40 viruses; discovered chlorophyll cells divide every 26 seconds.

*Technical** issues: 1930, Pasadena, Ca., Rife introduced the monochromatic lens; reference is made regarding a stethoscope Rife developed that attracted the interest of medical doctors. Rife worked on a special lens for three-dimensional motion pictures for a prominent movie studio; assisted an associate in development of a lens for automotive headlights to reduce oncoming glare so prominent in automobiles of the era; had capability to design and construct optical instruments to meet the needs of any capacity; had a research facility for salt water conversion in San Diego.

Miscellaneous: Rife played french horn for the San Diego symphony, played stringed instruments as well. Rife was honored for contributions to motor racing and high powered boat racing — 1900 to mid 1930's. (There is not enough information to clarify the issue of racing contributions.) Rife was a hunter, sportsman and enjoyed gardening. Rife constructed his own guns and fishing rods. (That would require expert engineering and craftsmanship!) 1969: Became member of Bahia Faith and helped form the First Spiritual Assembly Of Bahia's in El Cajon, California.

*Statements from associates indicate Rife did everything with pride, enthusiasm and perfection.

Special note must be given to the fact many of Doctor Rife's degrees were honorary. This is an important issue since many of Rife's detractors apparently ignored Rife's honorary degrees and placed their faith solely in degrees earned through the courses of accredited universities, specifically in the field of medicine. It must be pointed out that Rife did not have the opportunity for such extended education. He also may not have benefited from such education. Rife was in a class by himself, he found a 'niche' in the world of science that only he could fulfill. Perhaps such extended education might have encumbered his course and reduced his abilities to 'think freely' and attack problems without the dogma of specialized education and the associated narrow guidelines that go with it. As it was, Rife's detractors, men with degrees and great credibility (among themselves), simply could not accept someone 'below them' displaying such phenomenal creativeness and scientific discoveries. In reality, it seems Rife's technical and professional background was far superior and more advanced than most of the so-called 'professional' critics.

Professional jealousy, dogmatic skepticism, greed prevented a scientific genius from establishing true humanitarian goals and principles for the benefit of all!

In a document containing answers to questions which were asked of Rife to clarify the issue of professional background, Rife made the statement that, "The American Cancer Society was interested in his cancer cure until they found out that he, and Crane, were not medical doctors. Then, the proposed research project was stopped".

Other points of information relating to Royal Rife, according to his words, were that, at one time, Rife had one of the best 'privately' equipped laboratories in the world. The facility had a complete machine shop, million volt X-ray, glass blowing equipment, surgical instruments, sterilizers, pathology room, research animals, various microscopes, (some of which were Rife's own design). All forms of electronic testing equipment, frequency instruments, micromanipulator and other equipment. A stop motion microscope was set up for the life study of microorganisms, "from the cradle to the grave".

Rife described the procedures to filter and isolate viruses. He claims to have isolated viruses for: cancer, typhoid, tuberculosis, herpes, b-coli, poliomyelitis and about forty other viruses that had never before been isolated. He was able to culture these viruses at will. He could introduce a virus into a lab animal then eliminate the virus, returning the animal to normal health, at will, using his specialized procedures.

One test procedure was repeated **411 times** to prove that a virus was the causative agent of cancer. In his powerful scope, Rife saw "viruses released just as a chicken lays an egg".

Rife named some of the qualified people he had worked with: Milbank Johnson, MD, Arthur Kendall, Ph.D., E.C. Rosenow, MD, Coolidge of General Electric, O.C. Grunner, MD, Dr. E.F.F. Copp, MD, Alvin G. Foord, MD, Ernest Lynwood Walker, MD, Karl Meyer, MD, of The Hooper Foundation of San Francisco, George Dock, MD, Wayland Morrison, MD, Fischer, MD, James B. Couche, MD, Charles F. Tulley, DDS, Arthur Yale, MD, Hamer, MD, J. Heitger, MD, Royal Lee, PhD, T.O. Burger, MD, Dr. Ray Lounsberry, MD, Dr. Rufus Von Klein Scmidt, MD.

Technicians: Henry Siner, Verne Thompson, Ben Cullen, Phillip Hoyland, John Crane, Dave Sawyer, Agnes Bering, Alice Kendall (daughter of Dr. Kendall).

Dr. Milbank Johnson, a multimillionaire, set up and supervised three human research clinics. The first clinic was set up under a special medical research committee of the University of Southern California with Dr. Rufus B. Von Klein Scmidt on the committee, in the home of Ellen Scripps in La Jolla in 1934. (This was the facility where 16 critically ill patients were treated with Rife's Ray device. All were healed -- an amazing 100%.)

Per Rife's statement: "...And, the AMA has suppressed all effort and research knowledge of my developments."

COMMENTS:
Although court records indicate Rife had sold 'all' equipment and rights to Crane for ten dollars, other documentation indicates more finances were involved. Crane, and others, did purchase various pieces of equipment at various intervals. Nonetheless, the amounts paid were a mere fraction of true value!

Rife and Electronics:
There seems to be no information as to where Rife may have received education in electronics. Lee DeForest of radio and electronics fame and Rife were good friends and did work together around 1920—1921 which certainly was a good source of information for Rife. Although Rife was an obvious genius and a man of many talents, he could not have been completely versed in all (variable) fields. Also, one must consider the 'level' of electronics of the era. It is likely Rife had to rely on others for electronics applications, electronic equipment, frequency generation, design and construction. Electronics was a critical area in Rife's work and having to rely on outside assistance must have placed Rife at moderate disadvantage. Rife let it be known some technicians created problems for him. It appears Rife struggled somewhat in the area of frequency generation and application. Rife certainly had capabilities in electronics but to what degree? (This speculation will likely generate controversy!)

Although no evidence has turned up to indicate a direct connection between Rife and Nicola Tesla, it is a reasonable possibility. Evidence indicates Rife did have access to devices made by Abrams, Lakhovsky and Tesla. We know Rife did wind coils and certainly did construct much of his electronic equipment. But, he may not have kept pace with electronics through the years.

The following is an excerpt from correspondence to Rife from an associate in England dated 1939. **This is in reference to the 'scientific sun dial' previously mentioned:** "Your department of navigation is no doubt going full blast under the very capable direction of Professor Ashlock and his partner, Admiral Root. It will not be long, I am sure, before a universal demand is created for the instruments under construction. May good fortune and success be with you ever."

*San Diego Union, May 8, 1950: Conversion of Sea's Brine To Potability, S.D. Group's Aim: This article is in reference to Rife's suggested application of frequencies to knock impurities (elements) out of the water. With use of proper frequencies, selected impurities could be removed from the water while leaving desired elements in. Rife considered such a method might be far less costly than methods requiring expensive fuels to convert water through the distillation process.

*Photography and Rife: Rife was well versed not only in the optical requirements of photography but also film processing, motion photography and many other aspects dealing with film, micro-photography and general photography. Rife was often called upon by others to resolve issues relative to optical and photographic problems as related to medical and industrial research, the motion picture industry and other photographic requirements!

*San Diego Union, April 16, 1934: World's Biggest Microscope In San Diego. "A single blood cell occupies the entire field of the Rife microscope."

A few photographs on the following pages are designed to intrigue the reader to follow through with research of their own. Thanks is offered to the many Rife researchers who have taken time to dig up Rife artifacts and present them to interested parties.

For a website with true and extensive legacy of Royal Rife, complete with photographs and major historical documentation, see:

http://rife.org/index.htm

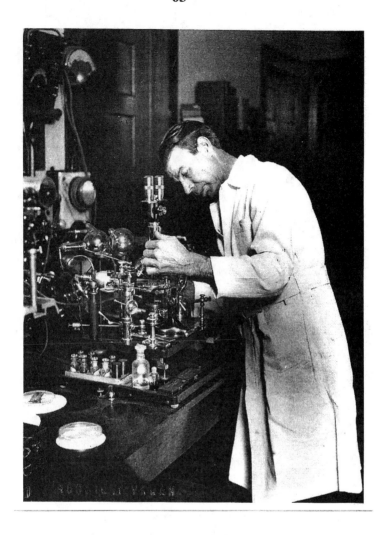

Royal Rife in his laboratory working with one of his prismatic virus microscopes. A double, bubble beam ray tube can be seen behind and slightly to the left. Rife stated this was the best tube of all. In movie film of Rife working in his laboratory a brief flash of the tube was all that was required to devitalize pathogens.
(November 2, 1929.)

Photo courtesy of San Diego Historical Society Photograph Collection - Union-Tribune Collection. (Copyrights apply.)

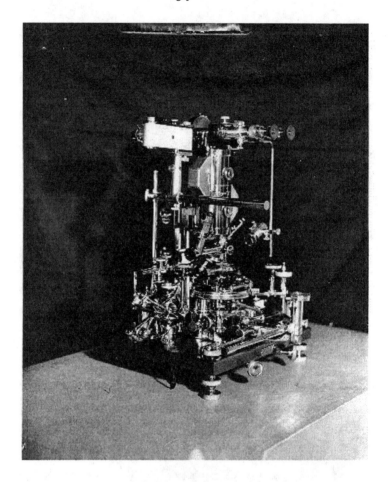

Rife prismatic virus microscope. Over a period of many years five such microscopes were constructed. Rife virus microscopes were extremely complex as was verified by a group of Rife advocates that seriously attempted the challenge of duplicating a Rife microscope. Camera mounted near top for photographic recording!
(November 2, 1929.)

Photo courtesy San Diego Historical Society Photograph Collection - Union-Tribune Collection. (Copyrights apply.)

Photo courtesy Lynn Kenny.

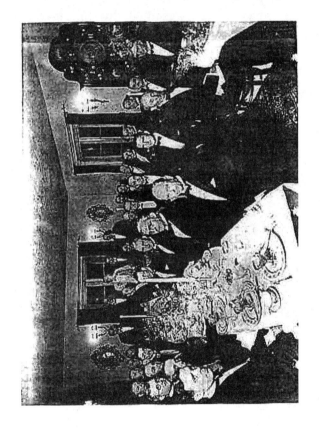

Photo plate adjacent page:
November 20, 1931

This is the 'famous' photo of Royal Rife and 'associates', at a dinner party given in the honor of Rife for his accomplishments and achievements.

The event was presented by millionaire, Dr. Milbank Johnson. Johnson was Medical Director of Pacific Mutual Life Insurance Company, President of Southern California Auto Club. He was also one of the political giants in the medical community. Many doctors at the event had participated in verification of Rife's work.

Years later, due to pressure from the AMA, many of the doctors, in attendance at the dinner, denied even knowing Dr. Royal Rife. In spite of Rife's wondrous achievements, the AMA later branded him a fraud.

One of the few doctors who continued to support Dr. Royal Rife, and who was to serve as a defending witness in favor of Rife in a critical court trial, purportedly 'died mysteriously' just prior to the trial. *Supposedly, as the result of an anonymous tip years later, it was learned the doctor **had not died of natural causes**.*

List of guests 'invited' to the affair:
Dr. Royal R. Rife (Guest of honor)

Dr. Arthur I. Kendall	Dr. Fosdick Jones
Dr. C.M. Hyland	Dr. Alvin Foord
Dr. V.L. Andrews	Dr. Milbank Johnson
Dr. Wayland Morrison	Dr. F.C.E. Mattison
Dr. Joseph Heitger	Dr. E.M. Hall
Dr. C.W. Bonynge	Dr. E.W. Butt
Dr. A.S. Heyt	Dr. E. W. Lanson
Dr. George Dock	Dr. O. Witherbee

(continued)

Dr. Harold Witherbee
Dr. Linford Lee
Dr, George Kress
Dr. Aubrey Davidson
Dr. Walter Breem
Dr. A.H. Zeiler
Dr. C.D. Maner
Dr. Allen Kanaval
Dr. J. Brandon Bruner
Dr. Rufus Von Klein Scmidt

Dr. B.O. Raulston
Dr. Albert Ruddock
Dr. Richard Winter
Dr. W.H. Sooins
Dr. C.E. ZoBell
Dr. R.W. Hammack
Dr. Ellis Jones
Dr. Samuel Tattison
Dr. Royal Lee

Also invited:
Dr. M. H. ZoBell
Dr. B. Winter Gonin
Dr. O.C. Grunner
Dr. James B. Couche
Dr. Arthur W. Yale

Dr. E.C. Rosenow, Sr.
Dr. E.F.F. Copp
Dr. Royal Lee
Dr. K.F. Meyer
Dr. E.L. Walker

Dr. Lee DeForest (Of electronics and radio fame.)

(*Spelling of names varies with documentation.)

Excerpts from photocopied letters. From Milbank Johnson, MD, Pacific Mutual Life Bldg, Los Angeles, California, to Royal Rife (San Diego).

10/08/1935: "We have tested the machine out very thoroughly both on animals and on cultures, and so far as we can see, it leaves nothing to be desired."

12/19/1935: "A meeting of the Special Medical Research Committee of the University of Southern California will be held December 26....."

(Page filler tidbits:)

SDUT 01/10/2001
Ex-senator appointed to $99,000.00 per year medical assistance post by a committee made up of former colleagues.

(California, November, 2000:)
A committee of appointed medical experts was formed 'to study alternative medicine'. No reference was given to any of the committee members being in the field of alternative medicine.

At an all day meeting to be held in southern California a specific late afternoon time period time was set aside for general public input.

Some naive members of the public did show up, only to find an empty meeting room — the entire committee had departed hours earlier.

Chapter Eight

Modern Medical Marvels

Americans are painfully aware of escalating health care cost as well as health care insurance which must keep pace. The rationale is the patient receives such marvelous care in the modern health system that there should be no need to explain or justify extreme high cost. The rationale may be correct; but, if the quality improves much more, along with subsequent escalating cost, only the wealthy will be able to afford such quality.

A news article declared that about 40% of bankruptcies were related to necessary but unaffordable health care.

Prescription medication is heading in the same direction. CEO's of pharmaceutical companies justify the high cost of prescription medication by expounding on the virtues of their wondrous product and cost of qualifying the products.

Competition among pharmaceutical companies has established a need for each pharmaceutical company to engage in unprecedented demands at creating and marketing new products on a production line basis. This alone is costly and possibly dangerous to public health.

Pharmaceutical companies and their related products have become critical factors in the stock market. The mere announcement of a favorable, pending new drug often causes pharmaceutical stock prices to soar. If the product later proves ineffective, as the case has been many times, the market value of stock shares plummet. Fortunes are made and lost in this arena! (CEO's of pharmaceutical companies earn millions in wages and stock options according to a commentary on television!)

The unfortunate problem with pharmaceutical drugs are the hazardous side effects which becomes a matter of weighing the bad side effects against the good effects. Side effects may be moderate, may damage organs; or, cause death! This can be a dilemma creating a situation of compromise which both patient and doctor have to deal with.

On the other hand, if there are choices through alternative intervention, then it should be presented to the patient as an option. But, this is not the way it is in our existing medical society. Instead of allowing patients the choice of alternatives, our system has laws to prevent application of alternative health resources. The laws are rigid to the point even conventional doctors, who know of useful alternatives, will not utilize them in fear of reprisal from the powers above them.

Chelation is a good example. Chelation is a viable medical tool, a simple procedure which is a slow infusion of a specific chemical formula into the blood stream. EDTA (ethylene diamine tetraacetic acid). This process offers a number of beneficial gains one of which is to rid the arteries and capillaries of material (plaque) that builds up, slowing or stopping blood flow.

If offered the choice, how many patients with clogged arteries would prefer to spend a few hours sitting in a lounge chair reading or watching TV while the IV drip clears the obstruction as opposed to the dangers and expense of angioplasty or open heart surgery? Yet, prospective heart surgery patients are not made aware of chelation because it is not considered an option by the modern orthodox medical system. Conventional medicine considers chelation a fraud and has made numerous attempts to rid the playing field of this unconventional, non-invasive process. Doctors are not allowed to consider chelation as a viable alternative;

yet, orthodox medical doctors might be found in the back room of a chelation clinic receiving treatments for themselves. This is one of numerous alternative possibilities that are looked upon in disfavor by the rigid dogma of modern medicine. (Compare mortality rates between chelation and heart surgery!)

Royal Rife offered humanity the choice of going through the rigors of medical treatment with toxic medication; dangerous surgeries; or, simply spending a few minutes in front of a glowing tube, killing off harmful pathogens. But, how many ill people were ever offered that choice? Medical doctors are not familiar with this phenomenal device; or, ill informed or intentionally misinformed. Reviewing the previously mentioned Clinical Research program, one should consider that Dr. Rosenow and associates would not possibly have jeopardized their highly respected reputations unless they had good reason to believe in what Dr. Rife had to offer. They must have had strong evidence beforehand that frequency treatment had something to offer or they never would have accepted the challenge!

Proponents of conventional medicine have the right to proceed in the manner they determine most suitable and productive toward their goals. At the same time, alternative medicine, treatments and devices should be equally available and not suppressed or dismissed. This is especially true for terminally ill patients for which conventional medicine has nothing to offer.

Fraud is the battle theme used by orthodox medicine against alternatives. But, how virtuous is orthodox medicine? News articles abound with tales of fraudulent billing practices, harm caused by improper administration of drugs, deaths during 'routine' surgery.

Medical Research:
    Is medical research really a glamorous and noble endeavor? Is it possible that certain medical programs are controlled much as lawyers selecting jurors for a court case in hopes of stacking the outcome in their favor? Funding of certain research programs seems to relate to the politics of the system. Researchers who paddle their canoe in an unfavorable direction risk intervention of funding. With such 'a hammer hanging over the head' a researcher may not be in a position to perform judiciously.

    A recent recommendation (1999), is for women who might be predisposed to breast cancer, to have their breasts removed to avoid the possibility of breast cancer. How can anyone top that? Several decades and billions of dollars spent in cancer research and this is the best they can come up with?

    Robert O. Becker's books, **Cross Currents,** and, **The Body Electric,** offers startling insight into this intriguing area.

    It seems (some) research funding is looked upon merely as subsidy. When we consider the unfathomable amounts of money poured into medical research programs over the past fifty years with little to show for it, we should be questioning what is really taking place. Periodically, great new discoveries are announced — then they seem to fade away. Could it be a way to perk up lagging interest in public financial contributions?

    Royal Rife, and later, John Crane, begged for funding in order to proceed with their work. And, this was well after they had documentation to prove their research was of value. Yet, they were completely ignored.

Chapter Nine

Fishbein 'The Great'!

Morris Fishbein: 1889 - 1976. Morris Fishbein received his B.A. from the University of Chicago in 1910 and received his M.D. in 1912 and was editor of the American Medical Journal of the American Medical Association from 1924 - 1949. (If the above dates are correct, Fishbein must have been a brilliant man: B.A. by the age of 21, and medical degree at age 23?)

Although the above records indicate Fishbein received certificates as a medical doctor there seems to be contradiction as to whether he actually put his qualifications to practice. However, it is known that Fishbein was editor of the JAMA (Journal of the American Medical Association) from 1924 - 1949.

Allegedly, by 1934, Fishbein held complete domination over the AMA. With the extensive influence of the AMA and control of the JAMA, Fishbein held the power to intimidate those who disagreed with his goals. He had the backing of politicians, lobbyists, pharmaceutical concerns, medical universities and wealthy individuals. His power was his most important asset which he used to successfully attack all forms of alternative medicine and related products! Perhaps he was justified in his course of action; but, that is for someone else to decide!

To digress, briefly, the internet, as well as municipal libraries, abound with information, past and present, regarding historical facts, people and places. Therefore, at this point, it is strongly recommended that the reader devote time to research of their own to gain a clear understanding of the influence and economics of modern medicine as a business monopoly. Specifically, the reader might take time to search the past and present history of: AMA (American Medical Association), in particular, Morris Fishbein, FDA (Food and Drug Administration); and, follow through with a review of the infamous attacks against Harry Hoxsey (1901 - 1974) of Hoxey Cancer Clinic fame, and Max B. Gerson (1881 - 1959). After reviewing the facts for yourself, the information to follow will become more understandable!

Harry Hoxsey had inherited the Hoxsey family formula which was a mixture of selected herbs that proved to be a formidable cancer fighting agent. Over a course of many years, Hoxsey opened seventeen clinics throughout the country, serving literally, thousands of patients. Hoxsey's success rate was more than the AMA (Morris Fishbein) could tolerate. Fishbein's initial attempt at intervention failed. This brought the wrath and power of the medical system against Hoxsey. Hoxsey became the target of investigations and harassment. Hoxsey was arrested over 100 times in two years.

For twenty-five years, Hoxsey and Fishbein engaged in ferocious verbal, media and legal battles. As often as they tried, the AMA could not prove Hoxsey's treatment to be fraudulent — there were too many satisfied cancer survivors. Eventually, a Congressional investigation sided with Hoxsey. (See the Fitzgerald Report!)

A prominent magazine editor sent a reporter to Hoxsey's Texas clinic to write a lengthy story covering the Hoxsey cancer curing fraud. The writer, James Wakefield Burke, was welcomed by Hoxsey. Burke spent six weeks investigating. Burke's conclusion was the Hoxsey formula was indeed saving lives, either healing or placing cancer in remission. Burke submitted his final report entitled: "The Quack Who Cured Cancer!"

In addition to charges made by the AMA that Hoxsey's formula was useless, the AMA also charged Hoxsey was taking 'victims' for their money. Burke found quite a different situation; as, according to Burke, Hoxsey often treated 'needy' patients free and even paid for lodging during their stay in the area. *As a result of the positive image presented by Burke, the articles were never run.* (Many years later, James W. Burke became publicity director for Hoxsey.)

In spite of the failure of the AMA to discredit Hoxsey, in spite of the thousands of Hoxsey cancer survivors who testified in favor of Hoxsey and his methods, the AMA/FDA was able to eventually put Hoxsey out of business by closing up all Hoxsey clinics, simultaneously - about 1958. This was done through harassment and absurd technicalities. At that point, Hoxsey gave up and turned the Hoxsey Formula over to his nurse/assistant, Mildred Nelson who opened a clinic in Mexico.

(Re: video documentary: "Hoxsey, How Healing Becomes A Crime!' ISBN 1-885538-76-6)
(1-800-283-6374)

Similarly, it has been alleged, that after Rife's refusal to accept 'business terms' offered by Fishbein, coincidental events took place: critical data and equipment components either disappeared or were vandalized at Rife's Point Loma laboratory; an arson fire destroyed the multimillion dollar Burnett Laboratory in New Jersey, just as scientists there were preparing to announce confirmation of Rife's work.

Similar battles continue to this day. A recent battle that extended for over a decade was that of Stanislaw Burzynski of the Burzynski Research Institute in Houston, Texas, versus the AMA/FDA. Another is the battle of Hulda Clark versus the AMA/FDA. (See internet for updated information.)

It is interesting, as well as a matter of irony, to note that the AMA, under the direction of Morris Fishbein, initially refused to accept, and even condemned, the notion that dietary programs or nutritional supplements should be an acceptable adjunct for health and the curing of disease. While, at the same time the JAMA was heavily endorsed and funded by tobacco interests, even after the morbid facts of tobacco and health had been established!

Medicine, Politics and Money: How many old timers recall ads displaying medical doctors smoking certain cigarette brands? The Cincinnati Post, July 23, 1946, entitled: "Light Up—That Cancer Rumor Is All Wrong!" The article states the National Cancer Institute said, "there is no evidence which would indicate that tobacco smoke is a factor in the cause of cancer."

And, do you recall those commercials: "More doctors smoke (XXXX) than any other cigarette!"?

Fishbein is gone but his legacy lives on. All forms of alternative products, medicine, treatments, including chiropractics and chelation, and so many others valuable aids are labeled 'quackery'! According to past and present orthodox medical science, there is no place for alternatives, 'the public should not be allowed a choice'! The apathetic public has failed to realize the pending impact on the future of the health industry!

Chapter Ten

Case History

My problems began with minor incontinence, irritation and discomfort in the urinary system. I had that condition for three years and during those three years the condition became worse. I did go to orthodox urinary experts. They did nothing for the irritation and discomfort. They did perform an ultrasound and biopsy to test for cancer. The first ultrasound did not reveal a cancerous condition. A year later it had become cancerous. Not wanting to deal with the problems related to radical prostatectomy, I looked for alternatives while 'treading water', so-to-speak, with the local urologists.

Although I was making monthly visits to the urologists, nothing was done about the inflamed urinary system. The urologist did not have an answer. He just kept pushing for what he had been trained for — surgery.

As the months went by and nothing was done (by medical doctors) to alleviate the discomfort, the condition became more aggressive, spreading to other organs. I soon had problems in my entire mid-section including kidneys, colon, digestive system.

Still hoping to avoid surgery I searched for alternatives. I experimented with herbs, various commercial concoctions, as well as some very unconventional approaches. Although I experienced considerable relief, which certainly was more than I got from the conventional doctors, the cure was to elude me.

The infection was depressing my physical condition in general. I was tired, mentally depressed, irritable. I had a difficult time keeping pace with my occupation. To make matters worse, on the advise of 'my urologist', I turned to hormonal therapy. In desperation, I followed the well meaning doctor's advise and took the drugs. That was an experience I wish to eradicate from my life.

Life changed for the worse. After a few months of continued use of the hormonal therapy drug, which I chose to do rather than face surgery, my personality and my appearance was altered. (I must state the doctor did not recommend extended use.) My face became ashen and wrinkled. In the mirror, I felt death staring at me. I became irritated and aggressive. I felt like smashing into cars in front of me on the freeway. For the first time in over three decades of marriage I was engaging in verbal disagreements with my wife. All I got from the hormonal therapy were miserable side effects with no healing benefit that I could determine. I was on a downhill slide.

In addition, and, I believe as a result of the hormonal therapy, I developed fibromyalgia. (This is a condition that feels like arthritis but isn't. The soft connective tissue is extremely irritated, burning, painful.) Month after month the fibromyalgia progressed, as did the urinary problems. By the eighth month the fibromyalgia had worked its way into my sciatic nerve at which time it became extremely debilitating — I could barely walk, sit or sleep. Each day was an endurance test!

I had gone to a rheumatologist for the pain of fibromyalgia. All that 'expert' could offer were antidepressant drugs and pain killers with no hope of cure, just 'mask' the discomfort. I refused the drugs. (At the time I was in contact with a young lady with fibromyalgia who was following her doctor's orders. She was no longer functional. I had no intentions of allowing myself to end up in such deplorable condition!)

With all the above problems and prostate cancer I was desperate for any form of relief from which orthodox medicine had nothing to offer other than monthly visits, pain killers and hormonal drugs. Or, radical prostatectomy.

Of course, there were always the wonders of modern medicine with continuous, invasive testing procedures which cost dearly and never seemed to add anything constructive in my health battle. Between my financial outlay and my insurance, money was going out at the rate of over $1,000.00 per month, with no beneficial gains and my general health deteriorating each month. Insurance covered part of the expenses!

My search took an interesting turn. I had known of Royal Rife and his frequency 'Ray' device from an article in a magazine many years earlier. As a result, when doing a web search, I saw a post in reference to Royal Rife which immediately caught my attention. With information I was able to obtain through a web search, I was able to construct an experimental, basic Rife type frequency device.

With the device I spent many hours 'scanning' for 'hits' which simply means, trying to find a frequency that would work for my specific problem which was prostate cancer. To my astonishment I hit upon a frequency that dispatched my debilitating fibromyalgia. A few weeks later I rid myself of the urinary inflammation I had been dealing with for over three years. In both instances the effect was within minutes. And, this was without any negative side effects what-so-ever! Ridding my system of fibromyalgia and the urinary inflammation did wonders. I regained my strength and returned to normal activities! Shortly after, I quit the urologist who was doing nothing for me!

I believe this doctor was doing the best he could while being forced to adhere to the confines of orthodox dictates. He was working to introduce cryosurgery (freezing of cancerous tumors) to our local medical community. Cryosurgery, at the time, was an 'unproven therapy'; although, the local medical hierarchy was allowing review of cryosurgery. *Invasive procedures are generally acceptable!* I considered cryosurgery as an option but not totally convinced. As in any form of surgery much depends on the expertise of the surgeon. There can be complications. Cryosurgery may require more than one application, (procedure)! Although, it appears to offer merit! (Surgeries are now referred to as 'procedures' — sounds less intimidating!)

After the unexpected recovery from my fibromyalgia, I decided to pass my good fortune to the rheumatologist who had previously advised me there was no cure. I should have known better! When I explained my good fortune and the marvelous results, all I got was a curt:" Is it repeatable?" I then contacted the host of a well known health watch website and passed on my good fortune to that person to counter his offensive attacks against the very remedy I found so effective. His reply, a childish (with rude intent): "Aren't you the lucky one!"

I then passed the experience to my 'good friend', my family doctor. He listened with interest, however, that was all he could offer. His medical protocol would not allow him to venture into 'unproven' territory. Accepting the challenge would have placed him in jeopardy with his medical status which neither of us wanted to become involved with!

Even though I was willing to serve as a test subject, I could not locate a medical practitioner willing to risk his license while assisting me! Without follow up laboratory testing, I was floundering and helpless!

In reality, my small prostate tumor was not a matter of concern. It had gone unchanged since it had first been analyzed five years prior. I do believe the alternative methods I tried had held the tumor in check. It did not bother me at all. It had been the other problems that were the cause of my depressed health.

However, not wishing to continue with the possibility of advanced prostatic cancer I did seriously consider what orthodox medicine had to offer.

The 'gold standard' of course was, and still is, radical prostatectomy (surgical removal of the prostate). Another was cryosurgery which is freezing of the tumor. Of course, radiation was another (orthodox) option.

Careful analysis indicates all have advantages and disadvantages. None of them appeared to be in my best interest. I continued with my research, herbal concoctions, various alternatives and continued use of my frequency healing device. The tumor remained unchanged. It did not regress or progress.

I was holding my own nicely and in control of my well being! Then, suddenly, due to circumstances beyond control (which could be cause for another publication) a prolonged bout with a contracted, 'flu like condition', triggered an emergency requiring installation of a catheter. I was now faced with radical prostatectomy.

Although my attempt at dispatching the cancerous tumor was a failure; I was elated with ridding myself of fibromyalgia and the urinary infection. Orthodox experts had done nothing regarding the urinary problem and advised me fibromyalgia was incurable. Two out of three was far better than what orthodox medicine had offered!

There are numerous case histories of correcting maladies, including cancer, with similar devices; so, we know it works! The problem is, these cases cannot be verified for fear of reprisal by opponents of Rife technology and alternative treatment in general.

*—An elderly friend who had conventional cancer surgery later had a recurrence requiring additional surgery. After the second surgery, tests indicated the cancer markers were still in his system. That person followed with frequency healing and the cancer markers disappeared. That individual remained cancer free and eventually succumbed to heart problems from old age!

*—Another elderly gentleman suffered debilitating cancer of the throat and tongue. His tongue had been removed as a result. Much later, in conjunction with orthodox treatments, family members turned to alternatives and did obtain a frequency healing device. No, this is not going to be a miraculous cure story; but, something beneficial did occur. The gentleman was too far gone for cure. He was in terrible pain and misery. The costly prescription pain killing drugs were no longer effective. In addition, the drugs caused severe side effects which added to his misery. **Although the frequency healing device was not able to do much for his advanced condition, it did offer considerable relief from pain.** Unable to speak due to the loss of his tongue, he was able to let his care givers know when he felt he needed frequency treatments. When asked if the device was helping, he would smile and give 'thumbs up'! This was pain relief without side effects!

*—A personal experience of mine occurred following a dental procedure. Several days after getting a tooth capped the area around the base of the tooth suddenly developed a nasty inflammation. It swelled considerably and was extremely painful. Initially I thought it would be short lived and didn't call the dentist. After three days, I realized it wasn't going to go away by itself. By that time the weekend had approached and assistance was not available. I decided to give my frequency healing device a try. Within an hour after application, the swelling was reduced and all pain disappeared. By next morning it was perfectly normal. No swelling, no pain, no trip to the dentist!

All this should be adequate evidence that further research of frequency healing should be augmented with serious evaluation. But, if Rife couldn't gain acceptance with all his creditable efforts, it's doubtful this bit of empirical evidence is of any importance to the existing medical community. They prefer to ignore it!

With recent developments and increased knowedge in plasma emission frequency healing technology, I now believe my cancerous condition could have been dealt with using Rife frequency healing technology instead of the 'Gold Standard' — radical prostatectomy!

Had Rife been left alone and received assistance from the medical community instead of harassment, the years of research that Rife so meticulously spent and recorded could have been available to mankind. Many who chose the alternative route, would likely be allowed a more agreeable conclusion to their medical dilemmas.

I have since discovered reference from Royal Rife indicating even Rife had trouble dealing with prostate cancer patients. Modern day researchers have had problems also. But, the learning curve has produced improved results.

One issue modern, orthodox medicine stills fails to accept or take seriously, is 'cause' and 'maintenance'. That is to deal not just with surgery of sick tissue; but, to deal with the cause of the problem, to try to prevent it in the first place; and, further, to try to prevent it from recurring!

***NOTE**: This is time to interject with an important and possibly, puzzling issue. By now, an astute reader may be wondering why the author claims to have rid himself of a couple of illness with a single frequency treatment; while, at the same time, it was noted, some of Rife's patients required many treatments over a lengthy period of time — some up to 90 days. An interesting issue!

The length of time depends on the condition of the patient and the type of disease. A large cancerous tumor contains a large mass of infectious pathogens. If the entire tumor is destroyed in one treatment, the large mass of debris (kill off) suddenly creates a serious and unexpected major problem of toxicity which the body must deal with. For a system that is already in a state of disrepair, and a diminished immune system, this can be hazardous. Royal Rife apparently had encountered and recognized this problem and found it best to destroy tumor tissue a layer at a time, with a few days rest period in between to allow the body to dispose of the debris and recuperate before another load is dumped into the system.

For illness of a lesser nature, this does not seem to apply. Minor health issues may not require this method and can be treated in a single session. The prompt restoration of two of the health issues I was dealing with did not affect my system negatively. As a matter of fact, in both events, the following day, my overall health improved dramatically. I assume this was the result of ridding my system of the negative factors of the prolonged related health problems.

It also seems frequency healing can trigger the immune system to become more responsive, causing it to become a more aggressive part of the healing process as nature intended!

Further development of this technology, as well as other alternative technology, has shown that a cleansing program may be required to assist in effective treatment and maintenance. Cleansing programs may possibly assist in strengthening the immune system. Again, this requires additional research to verify.

Using a plasma emission tube as an antenna, test subjects are generally in the range of four to fifteen feet. (I find seven feet works for me.) As stated previously, it is theoretically possible to treat a roomful of people at one time, indicating frequencies travel further.

This brings us to a interesting event. We had a visitor who stayed with us several months. The visitor brought a 14 year old cat into our home. The cat suffered from arthritis — **the cat had been limping badly for several years and was rather lethargic**. When I was running frequency programs for myself, the cat would often hobble to the entrance of 'my Rife room' and sit in the doorway for 'a visit'. **Within a month, it was noted, the cat was no longer limping, walking normally, had become active, even playful**. Cat and owner have since moved elsewhere.

Regarding this 'interesting event', I am sure the first sarcastic comments of 'an expert' will be: 'Is it repeatable?'.

Update: Well past the age of 19, the cat finally succumbed to old age. But, up to the end, the cat was active and walked without the noticeable limp she had prior to the stay in our facility.

Present day, orthodox, medical experts will firmly disagree with all this, which is their prerogative. They have been led to believe this technology to be fraudulent and label it quackery. This is unfortunate because it is real, it is effective. But, it does need further evaluation which no one should be allowed to prevent! However, the nature of research is important — it must be impartial and ethically supervised!

SCANNING:

To clarify the issue of 'scanning', it is a simple, although time consuming, process. Scanning is merely running a series of frequencies testing for results.

When this 'experimenter' did away with fibromyalgia and the long standing urinary inflammation, it was done through the process of scanning.

However, as an enthusiastic new Rifer and experimenter, the author made the mistake of randomly selecting frequencies and failing to record them. Thus, when the eight month old fibromyalgia suddenly and unexpectedly disappeared, although there was no question it was the result of the frequency treatment, the frequency was unrecorded and unknown.

An important lesson was learned — a method was established whereas frequencies are now run in orderly, sequential groups and recorded. A series of frequencies are run early morning; then, another sequence in the evening. Fifteen frequencies are run at three minutes each, over a forty-five minute time period. A record of the frequency series, duration, date and time are logged. The next segment begins where the last one left off.

A suggested approach is to begin at 20hz and work up in 10 cycle increments. That is, 20hz, 30hz, 40hz, etc. In the multi-digit range: 2,000hz, 2,010, 2,020hz, etc. It is suggested a beginner should avoid frequencies above 5,000hz. Interestingly, an amazing number of pathogens seem to respond in the low range from 20hz to 900hz.

Duration:

Duration is the length of time a frequency is run. Short duration of 3-minutes is standard protocol while scanning or searching for a usable frequency.

Some 'experimenters' feel a 'hit' although most don't. My reaction to a certain frequency was an initial agitation of my condition. It was then necessary to backtrack to determine which frequency caused the agitation. Once the frequency was pinpointed, that frequency was run for a longer duration. Sensation to the frequency was felt for 12 minutes, then suddenly stopped. At that moment realization set in. **An unbelievable 'devitalization' had taken place!** The 3-year old urinary problem had suddenly and immediately cleared.

The sensation could best be described as sloshing soda pop in the mouth — an internal effervescent effect. For this experimenter, it was the first and only time 'the ray' was felt. Two frequencies were noted but, since the first corrected the problem, the second was not applied. The frequencies were: 4100hz and 2050hz. 2050hz appeared to be the prime (strongest) frequency. (Note: 2050 multiplied by two equals 4100hz — an octave apart. This should prove the involvement of harmonics or partials.)

This was several years ago. Since then, many researchers have established similar results for other conditions!

Caution: the experimenter is the responsible party. It may be possible a frequency could cause tumor growth or some form of harm! However, this experimenter does not know of such an occurrence.

None of the above has not been substantiated by proper testing or by medical authorities and will not meet requirements of repeatability; and, perhaps, is a one-of-a-kind, incident! All I can say is, it worked for me!

(Page filler tidbit:)

SDUT 2/16/1995
Doctor with Alzheimer's left trail of errors:
A prominent physician practiced four years after being diagnosed with symptoms of Alzheimer's disease. -(Snip)- Hospital officials were careful not to infringe on a distinguished physician's rights.

SDUT 2/12/2001
Drug companies don't always reveal side effects in trials:
Researchers reporting on the effectiveness of new drugs tend to skimp on providing information on safety and side effects...

SDUT 2/22/2001
Baby gets liver transplant without blood transfusions:
A 7-month old baby received liver surgery without use of blood to meet requirement of parents religious belief. The medical team that arranged the special surgery were impressed with results and stated from now on they would use the same surgical techniques to avoid use of blood on future patients.

Chapter Eleven

Medical Testimonials:

The absolutely disturbing element of the Rife story is suppression, oppression, political pressure and outright and sadistic destruction of the work and findings of Royal Rife for which he devoted his entire life. Rife was undermined and persecuted along every arduous step of his phenominal research! Friends became enemies. Many associates were later to deny they had ever met or worked with Rife! Evidence of research programs and research documents disappeared. Those who attempted to remain true to Rife were faced with difficult times, with loss of their medical license and livelyhood.

In an interview taken of Rife by John Crane in the late 1950's, Rife made many statements that exposed the raw truth. In the early stages Rife had many supporters. Some were genuinely interested in the benefits of frequency emission healing. One ardent supporter was Dr. Milbank Johnson of Los Angeles, California area. Milbank Johnson was a multimillionaire and a powerful force in medical politics. Johnson was instrumental in the special medical research program held in San Diego in 1934 whereas Rife displayed the efficacy of his frequency instrument. A few years after the trials, Johnson died. With Johnson out of the way, according to Rife and his associates, the tide of medical politics turned against Rife and his marvelous healing device. From that time on Rife's path was a hazardous and discouraging struggle. The premature and unexpected death of Dr. Johnson, Rife's major supporter, was clouded in suspicion.

After the 1934 clinical trial, Dr. Johnson appointed Dr. James Couche of San Diego, to follow through with further investigation and research of the Rife frequency device and the two remaining patients. Dr. Couche had an extensive history in medical practice serving aboard naval ships and later, as a 'country doctor' in a rural area. Dr. Couche truly followed the doctrine of the Hippocratic oath - if the patient could not pay Dr. Couche took care of the patient anyway. If the patient was able to pay, that was a bonus. Dr. Couche held no fear of the medical community and proceeded as he saw fit which came to include extensive use of the Rife Ray device. When Dr. Couche attempted to join the medical association his application was rejected. Although he offered no proof, Dr. Couche was firm in his belief the rejection was the result of his use of the 'unapproved' Rife device.

Dr. Couche used the Rife device extensively for many years with "excellent results"!Ced Dr. Couche often successfully treated ill patients that had been passed unto him by other doctors who felt they were losing the battle! Hideous butterfly lupus was cleared up in several patients. Patients with destructive, life threatening diseases, including cancer, were returned to normal health, with tests results indicating all signs of cancer had left the body. Dr. Couche healed many cases of tuberculosis including his own son who had contracted the disease while in England. Dr. Couche used the Rife device on his wife as well as himself to keep his body healthy. Upon interview by Crane in the late 1950's, Couche stated that even though he was in his mid-eighties, he was in perfect health and attributed it to his Rife device!

Dr. Couche made the observation that a room full of patients could be treated simultaneously. He also commented that the intrument was a marvelous tool since treatments were painless and simple. When in doubt about a medical problem Dr. Couche applied the ray device since, "it could do no harm".

Dr. Tulley, also of the San Diego area, was a well respected and innovative dental surgeon. Tulley was introduced to the Rife device by Dr. Couche who successfully treated a chronic ailment Tulley had. Following the treatment Tulley obtained a Rife device which proved to be a great tool in his work. Dr. Tulley healed numerous cases of mouth and gum infections without surgery; and, where surgery was required, by treating patients with the device after surgery, patients did not develop infections.

Dr. Hamer was supervisor of a San Diego hospital. Dr. Couche cleared Dr. Hamer of his chronic sinus infection. Dr. Hamer became enthralled with the Rife device and purchased one for the hospital. Dr. Hamer began successfully treating patients who had failed to respond to orthodox medical treatment. Many patients no longer had to make return visits. The loss of patients infuriated staff members and Dr. Hamer was given an ultimatum: 'Get rid of the device or leave' — he left!

Dr. Hamer opened a clinic; and, with an assistant, was treating up to forty patients per day with excellent success.

Dr. Couche used the Rife device for over twenty years on 'thousands of patients'. Dr. Tulley, Dr. Hamer and other doctors throughout the country accounted for many hours of use on numerous patients. Dr. Rife researched with the device for thirty years. All agreed, there was not a single case where the instrument caused harm to patient or operator!

Dr. Hamer healed a patient of a life threatening disease. The patient 'spread the word'. Shortly after, the Rife device was 'derailed' by the AMA!

(Page filler tidbits)

Rife made a statement that patients who had radiation treatments prior to frequency therapy, did not respond well to frequency therapy. Rife also stated that he could detect radiation in organ tissue up to six months after radiation therapy; and, up to two years after radium therapy.

Chapter Twelve

Doctor And Patient

Doctor/patient relationship is a critical factor in our health. Don't wait for ill health or an emergency before lining up your family doctor. The doctor builds up a patient history file which could be important when major illness strikes, especially when a patient is taking more than one medication or has unusual medical problems. Besides, it gives the patient an opportunity to find out how they will fare with that doctor with time to find another if things don't work out.

Doctors are human beings. And, like all human beings, doctors are not created equal. It is of the utmost importance to be on a level with your doctor where you can discuss health issues. (Providing you wish to do so!)

I have the privilege of having an excellent doctor\patient relationship with my family doctor! At times we may disagree but we work it out mutually! However, there have been times when my doctor has had to send me to associates, some of whom apply intimidation and feel a need to control their patients. If I encounter such a doctor, I find no need to continue with that doctor! It's best for patient and doctor to part company. Patients have the right to ask questions but I have found many doctors don't believe in patients rights!

Blood Issue:

The issue of blood transfusions involves implications and consequences that can become a serious dilemma in certain situations! Medical practitioners sincerely believe in using blood (transfusions) as a necessary medical tool. Blood, as a medical utility, has developed into a multimillion dollar per year business. However, there are implications in blood use that even medical science prefers to ignore — blood as a substance is unique to each individual. In addition, contaminated blood has become a serious health hazard with world wide epidemic of AIDS and abusers of illegal narcotics along with other related problems.

In 1999, a lengthy news article detailed the issue of millions of dollars loss of blood supplies contaminated by improper handling and processing.

One look at the caliber of some of the individuals lined up at a blood collection facility to sell their blood should be enough to convince most people that accepting blood may not be a wise choice.

Many informed people prefer not to accept blood as routine. There are also members of certain religious organizations; who, because of their faith, cannot accept blood transfusions. Yet, orthodox medical doctors are adamant in their decision to force blood on a patient even to the extreme of obtaining a court order to do so. They often refuse to acknowledge blood substitutes and blood expanders that are safe and acceptable. Why? Because for decades surgeons have been taught to utilize blood transfusions as a routine procedure — 'for the welfare of the patient'!

The average surgery patient pays little attention, the patient simply accepts what the doctors tells them is best. They may not even realize they were issued blood as part of their surgical procedure. These are the kind of patients doctors prefer. But, for patients who refuse to accept blood transfusions, the issue may become critical.

My medical problem suddenly turned into a life threatening nightmare. An unexpected, sudden change in status developed requiring an uncomfortable catheter.

Afterwards, I had to locate a new urologist.

I filled out the usual medical history forms. When interviewed, the doctor dwelled on what I had been doing about my condition since I had known about the prostate problems five years prior. I explained that for a couple years I had been attended to by a urologist who did nothing for me except push for radical prostatectomy which I hoped to avoid. I could tell by the doctor's attitude it would not be in my best interest to tell him all the alternatives I had subjected myself to and the fact I had been doing well until a recent incident, yet to be fully understood.

After poking, probing, and testing, the doctor asked why I had come to him. I explained the emergency and that I didn't know what to do at that point. The doctor was very annoyed and finally advised there was little he could do for me, I had waited too long, according to him.

I left his office in a state of mental shock, with the understanding I was terminal and nowhere to go.

A fews days later, I called back to see what could be done in order to at least remove the uncomfortable catheter. The doctor failed to return my calls. It was several days before I caught him by accident. I had become a medical outcast; his attitude was that of a police officer dealing with a criminal! But, lucky me, after pleading, I was able to negotiate another appointment.

We discussed options. Basically, it was radical prostatectomy or nothing. At least we could get rid of the catheter then determine what to do after.

Then we struck an insurmountable obstacle — *the blood issue*! My decision was my personal choice, not based on religious views. When faced with radical prostatectomy I advised the surgeon I would refuse blood transfusions. The surgeon became indignant and advised me I had no choice in the matter — I would accept blood or die on the operating table. He went on to explain that to get around the blood issue we could store several units of 'my own blood' in advance. He further advised me that 'he would unhesitatingly use donor blood should my supply be inadequate'. He further informed me, that should I survive surgery, I would be facing follow-up radiation treatments. The prospects were grim, to say the least!

I quickly lost faith in that surgeon. I was told if I didn't like the arrangement I could leave; and, leave I did. I left with the understanding I was terminal, in misery with an uncomfortable catheter, with no one to turn to. At that point I figured I had nothing left except my dignity and I was determined to save that much of what I had left!

Although it may be coincidence, in attempting to find another urologist, I found not a single local urologist would accept me sooner than 8 to 10 months away, even though it was obvious I needed immediate assistance! That left me only with prayer! That turned out to be the answer. My wife contacted a religious organization with sources just for such blood issues. Within days I was on my way to another town where the staff had a completely different attitude and outlook.

Where credit is due, it must be pointed out, there is a (growing) minority of orthodox surgeons who have undergone special training to perform surgery in such a manner as to 'control blood loss' and retain as much of the patient's blood as possible.

That is exactly what I found. The facility had a 'team' of specially trained surgeons and assistants who had mastered what they term, 'bloodless surgery'.

According to the surgeon in charge, they had learned through years of bloodless surgery that their patients recovered quicker, with less complications and overall, the patient survival rate has been much better.

In addition, an analysis of my scans indicated my case was not hopeless after all. On the contrary, the prospects were excellent. I went through surgery without mishap. No blood was administered, I was back home within days; and, my operation was so successful radiation follow-up was not needed!

Once again this proves doctors are not created equal, and that applies to hospitals and clinics as well. It seems certain methods, thinking and administration of techniques vary from one facility to another.

There are blood expanders and developments in oxygen carrying blood substitutes that may be utilized to compensate for blood loss. But, once again, with specific surgeons; or, in many clinical facilities, dogma prevails. Therefore, it is up to the patient or their families to intervene, ask questions and clarify issues. Looking into the matter ahead of time as to how local medical facilities will handle the blood debate cannot be stressed enough. Becoming involved in litigation between patient and the medical system when an emergency occurs is a disaster both sides must avoid!

Reviewing the first analysis against the final outcome, I now believe the first doctor was administering his brand of punishment for my failure to accept the terms of orthodox medical dictates when I was led to believe I was terminal and would die unless I unquestionably followed his recommendations!

(Page filler tidbits:)

The Smithsonian Institution (USA) has documentation on the Universal Rife Prismatic Virus Microscope; but, unfortunately, not an actual microscope!

A museum in London, England possesses a Rife microscope although it is in storage and not available to the general public. It is believed to be a microscope that Dr. Gonin, of England used as a research tool. Dr. Gonin and Rife remained good friends until the death of Dr. Gonin. This microscope was constructed by Rife in 1938. Although in fair condition, it does not seem to be in operating condition due to missing components.

(Information on this scope may be available on internet.)

Chapter Thirteen

Memoirs:

Benjamin T. Cullen was a mechanic who had known Rife (and Timken) from Rife's earliest days in San Diego. Cullen was later to become one of the principal founders of United Polytechnical Institute, which later became Beam Rays Corporation. Benjamin remained a good friend and admirer of Royal Rife even after the disastrous Hoyland/Beam Rays litigation affair.

In his latter years Benjamin was interviewed by John Crane as to his recollections regarding Royal Rife. Here are some points of interest:

Back in the days when Cullen performed major engine rebuilding for Rife and Timken, Cullen recalled Rife would often bring a musical instrument and play for any available audience. Rife played stringed instruments and wind instruments. Cullen recalled an incident during which Rife put on a one man concert in Cullen's garage. Rife began playing his French horn with such enthusiasm and artistic temperament that soon the whole block of people, which Cullen estimated at about one hundred, listened in awe. When finished, Cullen stated there wasn't a dry eye in the crowd, as everyone was stricken with emotion at the performance. Cullen stated Rife had put his heart and soul into his music, as with everything he did.

Cullen describes how in the early 1900's (around 1913), Roy designed and built his own aircraft. That included Roy making his own engines, engine cylinders, components, carburetors and whatever was needed.

About Roy's associates, Cullen had this to say: "Dr. Hamer is a whipped boy — he doesn't say anything any more. He was very 'indoctrinated'!" Cullen then said, Kendall had moved to Mexico, depleted his finances and later returned to San Diego to live with relatives.

Cullen brought forth other interesting bits of information about Royal Rife:

* Rife built a single, camera lens with which 3D pictures could be taken.
* "Roy developed a means of testing polarity of the material in the tubes and by matching polarity of the filaments to polarity of the poles he was able to develop more high frequency power." *This was Cullen's terminology. In a taped interview, Rife also used the term—filament—which indicates polarization took place in one or more of the vacuum tubes and not the phanotron.*
* "Roy's frequency experiments often broke lots of glass in his laboratory or store house; glass vials and windows." (Does this support audio frequencies!)

Here is interesting information that brings Hoyland and Fishbein into the picture which brought the Hoyland/Beam Rays litigation into effect. This is information brought out by Cullen although some of it may have been speculation on the part of Cullen:

All members of the Beam Rays Corporation were given equal shares — 6,000 shares each. Even though, at that time, Benjamin Cullen had put the biggest financial share into the venture. But, according to Cullen, Hoyland felt he wasn't being given enough for his efforts and wanted a bigger share of the venture, which is one reason why Hoyland initiated legal action. But, there's more (as they say on those late night TV commercials).

Dr. Hamer was enthusiastic over results he was achieving with Rife frequency devices. Dr. Hamer was busily engaged in treating patients and passing the word to others in the medical profession. According to Cullen, Dr. Hamer was running an average of forty cases a day through his office. Dr. Hamer had purchased two frequency devices and had hired operators to run them. Dr. Hamer was monitoring treatments closely while building case files in support of frequency healing.

Among the cases was an elderly fellow from Chicago who had come for treatment of a terrible malignancy around his face and neck which Cullen described "as a gory mass". Within six months, the man was healing and all that was left was a small black spot on his face — and that was about to fall off.

Another success story was the wife of Commander Benjamin Harrison. Harrison's wife had severe breast cancer and was in poor condition. Dr. Hamer treated the woman and healed her.

Somehow word of these successful frequency healing programs had gotten passed on to Fishbein (AMA). Fishbein sent an attorney by the name of Aaron Sapiro to look into the matter. Without getting involved in uncomfortable transgressions, let's just say the following joined forces to wrest away control of Beam Ray and discredit Rife: Hoyland; attorneys: Aaron Sapiro/Eli Levenson and Fishbein. Shortly after, the lawsuit began.

Rife was called before the judge to testify but Rife fell apart under pressure of examination and couldn't handle the affair. A doctor friend of Rife wanted to avoid prescribing drugs to calm Rife and suggested Rife take a drink of liquor instead. Unfortunately, that instigated Rife's drinking problem which sent Rife into a downward spiral!

Years later, as Cullen recalled, Rife could not hold a job due to his drinking problem. Friends had gotten jobs for Rife at Convair, Rohr and Ryan (San Diego aircraft construction companies) but Rife's drinking prevented him from continuing with employment.

Initially, a Dr. (xxxx) had been instrumental in testing and promoting Rife's frequency device. But, as time went on, the doctor became a problem! At one point Dr. (xxxx) went so far as to make an attempt at taking over Rife's frequency device as his own. The doctor produced and sold an estimated fifty Rife (type) instruments.

The doctor was constantly tinkering with Rife's frequency instruments, making alterations that would cause the instruments not to function properly. (This was confirmed by a statement previously made by Rife.) In addition, it seems Dr. (xxxx) caused the death of several patients through his own negligence, then passed the blame off on the frequency healing device. At that point, Rife took the equipment away from the doctor. One point Cullen made special note of is that after Dr. (xxxx) found Rife had developed a drinking problem, "***Dr. (xxxx) would intentionally give Roy too much whiskey***".

Cullen made an interesting point of how Rife would sit at his microscope anywhere from twenty-four to forty-eight hours at a time, barely moving. For that task, Rife was rock steady with nerves of steel, as Cullen stated. Before doing so, Rife would carefully prepare himself with a workout program. Then, Rife would literally strap himself in the seat. Cullen's reference to seeing Rife at his instrument: "That is what I call one of the most magnificent sights of human control and endurance I've ever seen!"

An intriguing event was related as to how Rife may have saved the life of Mrs. Timken. Mrs. Timken had become extremely ill. Medical doctors were unable to determine the cause of her illness. Royal Rife made a careful analysis and discovered the cause was from food in her refrigerator that was poisoning her. After recovery, Mrs. Timken came to Roy and said she understood Roy needed money for some experiments he had pending and gave Roy $30,000. After that, whenever she wasn't feeling well she would go to Roy for frequency treatments.

*Note: It must be pointed out that the preceding interview and recollections were taken when Cullen was about sixty-nine years old. Years had passed, his recollections may not have been accurate. Cullen's terminology and nomenclature, in some cases was lacking, such as his description of the tube components.

Technical Issues:
Thumbing through the pages of historical data regarding Rife, Crane and frequency technology, one issue stands out, clearly — lack of stability.

It seems this problem prevailed through the years. Researchers would achieve marvelous results for a period of time, then, suddenly, the system would fail to produce much of anything. Even from one day to the next.

This seems to still be 'somewhat' true with our meager equipment and attempts at repeatability. It's not so much a failure of the technology; but, appears to be an inherent problem co-related to electronics and atmospheric variations and other surrounding conditions. Changes in atmospheric pressure, temperature, magnetic earth fields and other surrounding natural forces affect electronics in strange ways!

(Page filler tidbit:)

10-03-1944, Dr. Johnson Dies After Brief Illness:
Dr. Milbank Johnson, 73 years of age, died following a brief illness. Stricken only Saturday, news of his death will come as a great shock to the community.

From the article we learn Dr. Johnson had an extensive history in the medical field. He was a humanitarian, philanthropist and benefactor to many. He held membership in numerous organizations besides having founded organizations of his own. Dr. Johnson was a multimillionaire involved in many successful business ventures. Johnson was well established in medical, community and state politics!

Chapter Fourteen

Medical/ Political Persecution

Persecution comes in many forms. Royal Rife was persecuted directly by refusal of the medical system to recognize or even consider the importance of his Universal Microscope, plasma emission frequency device and the years of sacrifice required in documenting laboratory research and his amazing concepts.

Rife was persecuted indirectly by associates who led Rife's efforts astray and hampered progress. The Beam Ray/British venture was an example. A fiasco causing loss of time and creating a negative reflection against Rife's credibility.

In reference to a technician, per Rife: "(xxxx) was like many men with whom I have associated over a period of years. In short time he began changing the basic principles of these instruments according to his own ideas." This affected potential results!

Doctors, researchers, associates and 'higher medical authority' undermined Rife's efforts and progress.

Per Rife: "I later learned that Dr. (xxxx) had ideas of his own and would have somebody change the frequency instrument to suit his individual whims." The alterations would make the instrument non functional and would not produce results as they normally should have.

Rife insisted on personally testing each instrument before shipping. This included microscopes, frequency devices and other optical devices. Yet, shipments were often processed without Rife's testing and approval.

The biggest blow of all was the Scripps research program. Most of the associates involved in that project later denied Rife due recognition and turned against Rife, an obvious result of 'pressure from above'.
Such persecution helped destroy Dr. Royal Rife.

Dr. Robert O. Becker began his career as an orthopedic surgeon in 1956. Dr. Becker went into medical research and became a pioneer in the field of regeneration and its relationship to electrical currents in living things. Dr. Becker's research led to amazing discoveries in regeneration of tissue and bone healing processes. His finding should have opened the way for new forms of healing, especially in relation to damaged limbs and nerves. Yet, his efforts were ignored and even ridiculed by his peers. His is another story of crucifixion and torment when a medical researcher steps out of bounds. A story of plagiarism, professional jealousy, dirty tricks. And, how critical medical research funding is manipulated to control those who don't follow the proper road. His books, **Body Electric** and **Cross Currents**, are educational, fascinating and open new concepts in the functioning of the human body and the relationship to magnetism and electrical currents. It also opens a window to the politics of medical research, distrust of and by colleagues, professional jealousy and suppression of unfavorable research results.

Dr. Robert Becker's research led him to reveal the destructive influence (on the human body) from the government and commercially induced sea of electronic and magnetic radiation that our modern world is engulfed in. The truth of his findings appears to have been unpopular with big business and the military!

If all this isn't enough to raise one's blood pressure, then 'The Fitzgerald Report', certainly should! The Fitzgerald Report was submitted into the Congressional Record Appendix August 3, 1953. In the 1950's, Congressman Charles Tobey enlisted Benedict Fitzgerald, an investigator for the Interstate Commerce Commission, to investigate allegations of conspiracy and monopolistic practices on the part of orthodox medicine. This came about as the result of the son of Senator Tobey who developed cancer and was given less than two years to live by orthodox medicine. However, Tobey Jr., discovered options in the alternative field, received alternative treatment and fully recovered from his cancerous condition! That is when he learned of alleged conspiratorial practices on the part of orthodox medicine. He passed the word to his father, Senator Charles Tobey, who initiated an investigation. The final report clearly indicated there was indeed a conspiracy to monopolize the medical and drug industry and to eliminate alternative options.

To show the power, financial and political influence of the medical system, to date, nothing has changed.

Why should practitioners of alternative health be forced to fight legal battles? Why do victims of ill health have to engage in sordid, costly, time consuming battles while attempting to gain the help they request? They are fighting a losing battle. They spend their time, money and resources fighting a heartless bureaucratic system, using personal assets, while agencies of the orthodox medical system have access to unlimited amounts of tax payer money, funding from inside the medical industry and the power of the laws they have created for themselves!

The history of medical practitioners and medical researchers persecuted by the power of the medical establishment and its policy of protectionism has been well documented by many publications for decades. Much reference material covering medical persecution is available in libraries, bookstores and the internet.

Harry Hoxsey, as well as Max Gerson, were practitioners who played decisive rolls in the alternative medical arena. Other important figures were: Dr. Linus Pauling, Dr. Virginia Livingston, Dr. William F. Koch, Dr. Ernst Theodor Krebs (biochemist), and, more recently, Dr. Stanislaw Burzynski and Dr. Hulda Clark. They were among many who have suffered the wrath of the medical system by paddling against the flow.

As a result of their unorthodox and 'unproven' treatments they were hounded by the power of the medical system and labeled as frauds and quacks. Some were forced to leave the country and set up shop elsewhere, under more favorable political environments!

San Diego Union, April, 8, 1960: "Vista Doctor, Nurse Jailed On Fraud Count." The 79 year old doctor and his nurse were arrested on charges of conspiracy to cheat and defraud patients with a complicated electronic machine.

Doctor Leonard Chapman had received his degree 55 years prior. "When I found Doctor Chapman, I was dying from cancer", stated the nurse, "look at me now!" It seems the nurse previously had abdominal cancer and was successfully treated by the doctor's unorthodox and 'unproven' methods and devices. She then stayed on as a nurse.

Both were arrested. The 79 year old doctor was handcuffed and hauled off to jail and treated as a criminal. Until his arrest, the doctor was under the assumption any method that produced results was a suitable method. He was to discover he was not up to date. According to the doctor's wife, "the doctor was to learn that cancer cures were restricted to surgery, radiation and chemotherapy. Anything else was not legal!"

The doctor had been using the same, reasonably successful procedures since 1923. Suddenly, in 1960, his procedures were illegal. He appears to have been using an Abrams radionics device. It is also known the doctor possessed a Crane frequency device but there was no specific mention of it in the news article.

One should wonder what justifies such vicious attacks even against licensed practitioners who sincerely believe they are doing the correct thing? One should also wonder why unqualified statements can be accepted by the court from one side while, at the same time, ignoring documented evidence from the other side. (Refer to Crane and Koch trials via internet!)

KEY WORD SEARCH:
http://www.williamfkoch.com/tests/martyr/Marty.htm
http://members.tripod.com/hoxsey/ward.html
The Fitzgerald Report
Gerson, Max
Hoxsey, Harry
Clark, Hulda
AMA
Morris Fishbein
Burzynski, Stanislaw, Houston, Texas, see also, antineoplastons

(Page filler tidbits:)

SDUT 12/19/1999
....Veterans hospitals mistakes kill 700...

SDUT 05/26/1999
...opposition to vaccinations worrisome to physicians...

SDUT 10/08/2000
Employers face health insurance rate shock

SDUT 11/12/2000
Prescription drug use is up, prices are higher and those that need medication are least likely to have insurance coverage...

Disastrous medical bills play a huge roll in personal bankruptcies in the U.S. accounting for about 40% of bankruptcy filings...

Chapter Fifteen

Miscellaneous Data:

The Evening Tribune, San Diego, California, 5/11/1938:'Rife Bares Startling New Conceptions of Disease Germs And Their Activities'. (This appears to have been a press release based on an interview with Rife. The writer was Newell Jones.)

The text of the article announces three new revolutionary conceptions of disease germs and their activities as disclosed by Royal Raymond Rife. According to the article this information was based on years of Rife's scientific research into the mysterious realm of the microscopic world of organisms.

Rife expands upon an apparent previous report of his as to the isolation of previously unseen, filter-passing viruses. Rife goes on to tell of the discovery of many kinds of previously unknown virus structures and views them as living entities rather than merely chemical constituents as previously suggested. Rife states the viruses appear to play a roll far greater than previously considered.

Rife explained the viruses have more forms of their respective kinds than previously known. He also announced that the organisms radically altered their fundamental biological characteristics after being fed different substances where they actually changed from one form to another within the same kind.

(NOTE: The change was labeled pleomorphism!)

This information followed his previous announcement of the discovery that tuned radio waves will kill disease causing organisms. Rife then discussed improvements of his high powered microscope. However, Rife, being the cautious researcher that he was, stated he was not yet ready to claim cures for diseases through radio waves. **(Remember, this is 1938.)** He felt more data was needed. Rife did state that his microscope, bacteriologic research and radio wave research were all linked together, helping make each other possible.

Rife said his most astounding finding was the alteration of organisms from one form to another. His research revealed that bacteria, and viruses associated with them, the small filter-passing, poisonous agent somehow linked directly with bacteria, are considered to be more direct, inciting cause of disease. And, that larger organisms can be altered by changing the media in which they are cultured in the laboratory. The organisms exhibited changes in metabolism much the same as man's consumption of oxygen — according to Rife's research.

Rife commented that these changes might explain why bacteria can be present in the human body without harm and then suddenly, cause illness. This, he theorized might result from some form of metabolic change in the human body which in turn causes a corresponding alteration of the bacteria, resulting in a harmless bacteria to become harmful.

Rife explained the case of bacillus of tuberculosis. Rife claimed the alteration to be so radical as to actually change from one form to another. In this case, the organism changes from a bacterial plant to a fungus, to a microscopic form corresponding to a visible plant life mold.

Isolation of filter-passing viruses was one of the most important steps in Rife's research which took years of exhaustive effort.

Rife stated he worked seven years straight and studied 20,000 cultures searching for a cancer virus, finally suspending the search since he had found nothing. Rife was later joined by Dr. Arthur Kendall, head of the department of bacteriology at Northwestern University Medical College. Dr. Kendall suggested a culture medium which proved to be the secret to success as Rife was able to press on and did eventually discover and isolate the cancer virus.

The culture was a mixture of pig intestine and tyrode solution. With this medium, Rife was able to isolate and identify viruses: b-coli, the seemingly harmless bacillus, which always seems to accompany the harmful typhosus bacillus, (according to Rife), tuberculosis, sarcoma, infantile paralysis, streptococcus and staphylococcus, herpes encephalitis and encephalitis lethargic.

Later, the renowned Dr. Milbank Johnson cooperated in the research program. Rife and Johnson, then found small oval motile, turquoise-blue bodies. This was reported in the California and Western Medical Journal, December, 1931. They surmised that these turquoise-blue bodies were the filter-passing forms of bacillus typhosus.

Typically, critics, 'the narrow minded medical experts who had not been involved in the research, but who knew all there was to know', attacked the findings, attacked Rife and Rife's microscope and his associates.
That brought additional help to the fray. Dr. E.C. Rosenow of Mayo Clinic's bacteriological department, joined the study. According to Dr. Rosenow, the oval motile, turquoise-blue bodies described by Rife and

Dr. Kendall were demonstrated unmistakably. **This was reported in The Proceeding of the Staff Meetings of the Mayo Clinic, July 13, 1932.**

Rosenow additionally reported that he, Rife and Kendall, later found filter-passing bodies from streptococcus cultures which might be the viruses that incited agents of infantile paralysis and herpes encephalitis.

Rife explained that the Kendall medium made it possible to produce filter-passing forms for study. This he theorized somehow caused the bacteria to assume a 'transitional state' allowing the shedding of smaller bodies which are viruses. Then, by means of the Universal Microscope, the particles could be made visible for study.

It becomes more intriguing when Rife claimed neither the microscope nor the medium alone were sufficient to reveal the filter-passing organisms that Rife had found in cancers. It was an unusual incident that made it possible. Rife had a tube of cancer culture which he accidentally 'rested' within a circle of a tubular glass ring of argon gas activated by an electric current. It was left 24 hours. Rife noted a change in appearance that attracted his interest. Shortly after is when Rife discovered filter-passing red-purple granules. Further experimentation proved these granules produced tumors typical of cancer.

Rife commented that this special illumination (under his scope) reveals the filter-passing organisms in individual, characteristic colors. He stated that no two kinds or forms of organisms have been found to have the same colors. **However, one form was found to have dual colors. The center portion of the rod form responded to one frequency while the ends responded** to another. **This required dual frequencies for devitalization.** According to Rife, if a single frequency was applied and that portion of the organism was devitalized, it would release the other constituent. Depending on which constituent was devitalized, either nothing would happen or the patient would die!

"It was found that by using combinations of these frequencies for different microorganisms that many other disease could be helped like sinus, ulcers, cataract, arthritis, poliomyelitis."

Another intriguing discovery made by Rife was polarization of microorganisms. Under the scope, if polarity was applied, the constituents would separate to the poles; a portion to the negative pole, a portion to the positive pole. Neither would culture individually; but, placed together, they would culture into a microorganism structure. As Rife put it, sort of, "male, female"!

Another important discovery was the pH factor. (Acid-base balance.) Rife stated if the pH was neutral he could not produce a culture. But, if the pH was altered to either base or acid, it would culture. Based on this information, Rife felt that if the human body remained in a neutral pH state, it was impossible to develop a disease.

Rife stated viruses to be a group of chemical constituents which could be altered by applying specific chemicals, parts per million, creating different organisms. By applying the proper chemicals, Rife could alter a given microorganism into a specific pathogen, at will, and back again; as long as they were within a specific group, of which Rife had identified about ten groups at that point.

Inoculation of experimental animals had demonstrated the disease causing properties of each virus isolated, according to Rife!

Correspondence from Milbank Johnson to Rife, 1935:
"Now that we have a machine in which we can give two frequencies at one time, it would be easy to treat all forms of tuberculosis both for the tubercle bacilli and *Much's granules.*"
(*Granules in sputum from TB patients, possibly degenerated tubercle bacilli. Re: Dr. Hans Christian Much.*)

Miscellaneous documents:
Rife: "I studied leprosy and I isolated a virus which we jointly demonstrated was common to rat, soil, and human leprosy and I found a frequency which would eliminate leprosy."

In reference to viewing microorganisms:
Rife: "First there must be high enough power to enable the observer to see them (viruses) and second they must be identified by a frequency of light which coordinates with the chemical constituents of the virus or filterable form in question. To my knowledge there is only one instrument today which will even show the viruses and that is the Rife Prismatic Virus Microscope which I built for this work. The electron microscope is a useless device for this study because the virus are killed instantly and you don't know what form you are seeing them in and they generally appear as round balls of dried up chemical particles."

Rife: "I saw Dr. Couche's brother who had come over from England. He had a 30 year sinus condition with terrible drainage. Dr. Couche used the frequency instrument on him and he was well in three weeks. Dr. Couche had treated Dr. Hamer, MD, for a sinus infection which cleared up."

Rife: "I saw cancer and tuberculosis cases that had completely recovered."

Rife: "Dr. Couche had treated Dr. Butterfield, MD's, brother-in-law who had a stiff wrist, a tuberculosis of the bone which cleared up. I also saw a Mexican boy who had osteomeylitis of the bone which Dr. Couche cleared up with the frequency instrument. I saw George Lemm being treated by Dr. Couche for tuberculosis and he had come out from Chicago to die. Lemm completely recovered."

The following is an excerpt from a letter written by a medical doctor in response to a woman requesting information on a frequency device she was considering for her husband. It is unclear as to what device; but, at the end of the letter the doctor suggests the woman contact John Crane in order to obtain a Crane device. (1960.): "Dear Mrs.(xxxx): We've been investigating the Rife Electromagnetic Therapy machine here in Dayton for the past 3 years. Our work has been primarily with cancer. However, I have used it on several persons with fungus infections of the feet (athletes foot). The results in the fungus cases have been most spectacular. - (snip) - After using the machine in rat experiments and on over 60 people, I feel I can tell you that it is definitely a safe procedure and will not hurt your husband."

In reference to treatment of eye conditions and cataracts it seems a temporary research clinic was setup to test Rife's frequency device. Here is an excerpt of a letter from one doctor to another doctor, dated June 1, 1937: "We treated the 'dewy' cornea condition empirically with the same MOR that we used on the cataracts and the dewy condition disappeared very promptly.- (snip) - Every case we have treated, with the exception of one which was a traumatic cataract where the lens was absolutely opaque and of recent origin, has benefited. The process of coagulation has been stopped and there has been a distinct retrogression of the opacities resulting, in most cases, in a complete restitution of the function of the eye."

Letter from a San Diego dental surgeon, Dr. T.... to John Crane, June 1, 1954:
"My first definite investigation was in that of my own case of prostatitis. A qualified urologist gave me (numerous medications) but the drugs did not do the job. The frequency instrument healed my case quickly. I then used the frequency instrument on a friend who was being rushed to the hospital for a prostate operation. He is perfectly well today without any operation or further medical aid. - (snip) - I had a case of butterfly lupus sent to me by a medical doctor friend and though it had been treated extensively and by specialists, the condition was large and in progression. After three months treatment with the frequency instrument the butterfly lupus disappeared. Another cancer case (carcinoma) was submitted to me for treatment with the frequency instrument by an M.D. friend of mine. He had an impossible condition but the frequency instrument dried it up in six weeks. I have found the frequency instrument very effective after surgery. I use it alone instead of antibiotics and have not had a case of infection. I have cleared extremely bad cases of trench mouth and pyorrhea in a few treatments with the frequency instrument. In conclusion I must state that I feel the frequency instrument is worthy of further research and that subsequent investigation and use will be of great benefit to all mankind."

The Case For Audio Frequencies:

Among researchers of Rife technology, debate continues regarding the issue of audio frequencies. Here are statements from Rife taken from an interview which took place in Tijuana, Mexico. (There is unfortunately no date on this document. But, it must have related to the John Crane trial of 1960/1961.)

"Initially, I (**Rife**) worked with loose couplers to get an audio oscillation and then with the use of transmitters I tried to balance the audio and modulate the audio on a carrier wave to transmit the audio energy. But, I found that both the audio and the audio transmitted through a tube as an antenna worked equally as well in a painless and harmless method to human tissue."

In the Crane trial we find: "...virus organisms could be devitalized or killed by audio frequency emitted from a device known as the 'Rife-Ray Tube'."

The Case For Square Waves:

This is still a topic of debate. None of the documents clarify this issue. However, from the viewpoint of electronics experts, it appears to be the most effective!

More On pH:

By use of electrodes in a solution, pH content can be measured. Therefore, pH level may play a role in effectiveness of frequency healing as well as other phases of healing. (Electrolytes!)

(Page filler tidbits:)

The San Diego Union, November 3, 1929
LOCAL MAN BARES WONDERS
Making Moving Pictures of Microbe Drama

Excerpts:

"R.R. Rife, Point Loma scientist, is photographing the hidden secrets of the microbe kingdom."

(Several photographs are shown including Rife operating his 'cine-micrographic camera, which he built to take movies of microbes'. A photograph is shown of a lock-jaw bacillus enlarged 217,000 diameters, which was said to be a world record enlargement.)

"The Rife Refractometer, has unparalleled flexibility for measurement of bacteria, parasitic organisms or the prismatic angles of crystals."

"The Rife experiment on the weight of bacteria which established the weight of a single average specimen at one-third billionth of a milligram."

"Rife is an expert in more lines than the average man has time to dabble in. He is an able bacteriologist, embryologist, electrical and scientific engineer, metallurgist, chemist, micro-photographer and he plays with scientific crime detection. As recreation he takes to target shooting of a half inch bull's eye."

Chapter Sixteen

Mamie Ah Quin Rife

Ah Quin was born December 5, 1848, in a small village in the Toishan District of Guangong Providence of Southern China. Ah Quin was the eldest son of a farming family. He had a brother and sister. Ah Quin's family relocated in Canton (Guangzhou), the provincial capital. This gave Ah Quin exposure to western culture since Canton was the only seaport in China available for trade with the west. Canton played a major roll in the emigration of Chinese to Southeast Asia and America. Ah Quin was able to take advantage of an opportunity for western education at an American Missionary School. He learned to read and write in English and Chinese and was exposed to Christian teachings.

The opium wars created economic upheaval leaving many Chinese families in distress. His family elected to send Ah Quin to the west, to the gold fields in America where he could make his fortune and hopefully send money to support his family back in China. Ah Quin was able to get to America where he spent several years in San Francisco.

In 1873 he was sent to Santa Barbara where he learned business and merchandising from an uncle.

Around 1877, Ah Quin began to accept western customs making many American friends along the way. He also began a diary which he kept up for over twenty five years.

In Santa Barbara Ah Quin became an employee of E.J. Gourely and Stearns. They had coal mining interests in Alaska which gave Ah Quin the unusual opportunity of a trip to Alaska where he was to cook at a company mining camp.

A year later Ah Quin made a brief trip to San Diego and from there back to San Francisco. In 1880 Ah Quin was offered an opportunity as a labor broker for railroad construction in San Diego.

Ah Quin set up shop in a business district in San Diego. In addition to being a labor broker, he also set up a business importing Oriental goods.

Ah Quin took time out to marry and eventually raised twelve children. In the meantime his business ventures flourished. Slowly he accumulated land and became a prosperous land owner with interests in other parts of the state.

Ah Quin was well known, a man of intelligence with a good western education. This allowed him many other opportunities such as being an interpreter in local courts cases involving Chinese who could not speak the English language.

To add to his business interests, Ah Quin became somewhat of a 'gemologist' which led him to become partners in a pink tourmaline mine in southern California which developed into a very lucrative venture.

Ah Quin was one of the first to install plumbing in his home in the Chinese district. Ah Quin encouraged the Chinese Community to improve their living conditions by setting an example!

Mamie, one of Ah Quin's daughters, married Royal Rife in 1912. Ah Quin died as the result of being struck by a motor vehicle, February 8, 1914.

The history of the Ah Quin family may not play an important roll in the life of Royal Rife. But, it is presented as a matter of filling in missing details to Rife's past in hopes someone might turn up more information that may become a valuable asset to the Rife legacy. Ah Quin kept a diary — is there anything in that diary or, someone else's diary that might shed light on some of Rife's long lost secrets?

A very nice monumental stone dedicated to the remembrance of both Royal Rife and his wife, Mamie, suggests the final resting place and monument were (possibly) a tribute from the Ah Quin family! (Since it has been noted Royal Rife died in poverty!)

**Credit is given for the preceding information that came from the Chinese Historical Society of San Diego. Special thanks to Murray K. Lee of San Diego, who in turn gives credit to a 1979 thesis written by Andrew R. Greigo, and to the descendents of Ah Quin and articles from the San Diego Union.

Rife's beloved first wife, Mamie Ah Quin died in 1957. In 1960, Rife married Amelia Aragon. This was probably during the period Rife lived across the border in Mexico. Rife documentation exists across the border but gaining access has been frustrating. Some old 'Rife style' plasma emission units, are purportedly still in use in Mexico, along with modern versions including pad devices and very sophisticated, electromagnetic units. Doctor's in Mexico still use the old rule — what ever works!

On the outskirts of San Diego, gold, silver and gem mines were once in abundance. Julian, California shipped several million dollars worth of gold and silver during its peak period in the late 1800's and early 1900's.

Ah Quin was a wealthy individual with a wide variety of business interests. Among his holdings was a mine in Ramona, California, not far from Julian. This was a pink tourmaline gem mine. Chinese favor gem stones of many varieties. Apparently, this mine was inherited by Mamie Ah Quin Rife. A San Diego resident expressed interest in purchasing the mine in 1937. It may be possible the sale of the mine was a result of losses Rife incurred in the Beam Ray Company fiasco although no specific mention was made regarding that aspect.

Chapter Seventeen

Frequencies and Theories!

A frequency, Mortal Oscillatory Rate, (MOR) is generated which excites an object — for our purpose a single cell microorganism. If the proper resonant frequency is applied and if the induced vibration is powerful enough, continues long enough and rapid enough, it will disintegrate the microorganism. This is a basic and simplified application. This has been proven and displayed on film. However, the scope of frequency application goes well beyond such simple destruction.

Theoretically a malignant microorganism, which, after being radiated with the proper frequency (MOR), may not necessarily be destroyed but converted (mutated) into a benign structure. Rife had proven that a virus could be altered (mutated) from one form to another by altering its chemical constituents. (A few parts per million.) Thus, by utilizing resonant frequencies of the chemical components, Rife felt he could mutate the microorganism at will!

Of course physicists apply theories relative to the complex issue of cellular structure, molecules and electron displacement which is all well beyond the scope of this publication. Suffice it to point out that Rife frequency healing research has proven to be effective, without harm to surrounding tissue, organs, bodily functions!

Reference, the Microscope and Light Frequencies:

An intense needle point of light is passed through the condenser lenses and up into the optical system of the microscope. By precise manipulation of specially designed quartz prisms a frequency of light is produced that is in coordination with the chemical constituents of the virus being observed. According to Rife: "although this appears to be polarized light, it is not." The light frequency is segregated into the desired mono-chromatic light beam. A frequency of light is found that displays the virus in its true chemical colors after which the predominant chemical factor can be isolated.

More on Dual Frequencies:

Rife proved a virus can mutate from one form to another by altering chemical constituents and creating virus mutations. Here we again find reference to **dual frequencies**! As stated by Rife: "I worked a great deal on tuberculosis. I isolated a virus from tuberculosis which I consider similar to what has been heretofore known as the poison molecule of Vaughn that had been isolated many years ago. He (Vaughn) did not isolate the organism, he isolated a chemical particle." Rife goes on to explain: "I finally found a MOR that would kill 'these' bacteria. I found the MOR of the virus of tuberculosis and also the MOR for the rod form. If the two frequencies are used simultaneously or one after the other, over the same carrier wave, the patient gets well. If only one of the frequencies is used you either kill the patient or accomplish nothing."

The reason for the above, according to Rife's explanation is, if the bacilli of tuberculosis is killed, a virus, the 'poison molecule of Vaughn', is released which reacts with the dead bodies of the rod form and produces toxemia and death.

Other Issues:

Each pathogen or virus has a frequency of its own. A healthy cell has a frequency; but, when that cell becomes contaminated or altered, the frequency is altered.

That is one reason why frequency treatment can safely be applied. The correct frequency will affect only the unhealthy cell, or diseased tissue, while leaving healthy areas untouched. Rife proved this beyond doubt. Still the closed minds of higher medical superiors would like us to believe frequency healing is unsafe.

Selecting proper frequencies (MOR's) continues to be an obstacle in Rife research. However, researchers are working on the problem. The basic method is trial and error. However, a recent scientific approach holds promise. This involves genome research requiring scientific expertise. In some cases the responses are very accurate. This method is under serious investigation and is under patent.

In some cases, frequency treatments result in virus destruction and rapid recovery. In other cases frequency healing appears to work by alerting the depressed immune system to become more aggressive, thus causing the immune system to attack the disease as nature intended. This is a slower process.

Before we proceed I must reiterate, I cannot claim this treatment to be totally devoid of hazards or that it is a cure all. For some, it may not work at all! I am not a medical doctor and I am not an electronics expert. What works for one person, may not work for another. I can only state that I 'experimented' with frequency healing and did eliminate 'my' fibromyalgia and a chronic three year old, urinary infection. Neither of these conditions was curable by orthodox medication or treatments. I took it upon myself to deal with the problems and was fortunate to be successful and without side effects! But, that should not imply that it will work for others equally as well!

Although my attempt to eliminate a cancerous tumor was not totally successful, I must point out overall results were a success rate of two out of three conditions. Certainly better than the odds I faced with the orthodox system. If orthodox medicine had no cure for (my) less complex issues, how could I have faith in their method of dealing with more difficult issues — like cancer? Additionally, I must clarify the device I was able to construct was not a true replica of the device constructed by Royal Rife. No one knows for certain how his device was constructed or why it was impressively successful. My version was a low cost experimental device; but, reasonably effective!

We also lack the advantage of Rife's Microscope which held the key to success. Rife scanned with generated frequencies while monitoring the effects through his Universal Microscope in order to pinpoint the mortal oscillatory rate (MOR's) required to dispatch the offending microorganisms.

Rife stated his device offered some 14,000 possible frequencies. Some must be exact (fundamental frequencies) while others work suitably as long as they are close to the desired frequency (harmonics or partials).

One problem Rife did not have to deal with is power restriction. In the modern world we are forced to operate with less power than that of Rife's device in order to avoid conflict with FCC regulations.

Frequencies must be transmitted to the desired location. One method is to radiate a given frequency through air, as from an antenna. Another method is direct contact. Rife used the first method!

The radiant method requires a transmission band, (carrier wave) radiated through the air. The carrier wave is then used to transmit frequencies to the target.

The subject is not physically connected to the device — frequencies travel through the air. It is effective when done properly.

Rife utilized a phanotron tube as an antenna. His preference seemed to be helium gas. Other noble gases also serve well and each has different characteristics which have yet to be fully examined. This may be referred to as '**Radiant Plasma Emission Technology**'.

Technically, a radiation device could be used to treat multiple targets within the range of the field. For example, treating many patients within a room, all at the same time.

A disadvantage of such a device is possible conflict with Federal Communications Commission regulations. The FCC is a reasonable group but they have their job to do and we certainly wish to maintain good terms with them by abiding to their regulations. Experimental and research work is confined to a limited band range. With rapid developments in electronics and communications, the FCC is in constant battle over issues of designating and controlling wave bands for the never ending demand of new applications.

The second method is more simplified. A frequency generator coupled to the target with some form of contact pads or coils and wires connected to the frequency device. These are contact devices. These devices are generally not in conflict with FCC standards. One possible disadvantage is the required current flow used to 'carry' the frequency wave. The other is a common law of physics: electricity travels along the path of least resistance. In simpler terms, the 'skin effect'. This means the current may tend to follow the path of the skin, possibly a vein, or the surface of an organ, which may cause the frequency to by-pass the intended target. Still, contact devices have proven to be effective.

Other Healing Applications:
Diathermy, (heat), is another method of dealing with cancerous tissue. This method has been successfully used in Europe. This system requires a method to generate heat in specific areas. Temperature is critical. This certainly is not something an unskilled person would experiment with. The opposite, freezing of tumors, has been used with some success but also must be carefully controlled to avoid damage to surrounding tissue.

Extremely low electrical currents appear to have been successful in dealing with certain illness like AIDS.

Another device under experimentation uses magnetic fields via coils that surround the target. This is being investigated for arthritic problems.

Yet, another system uses a somewhat more sophisticated version of Rife's device. Scientifically, it is termed a 'frequency-modulated, pulsed electromagnetic field' device. According to the developers of this system, the body can be scanned for cancerous areas followed by destruction of the cancerous cells. Basically, the device identifies the frequency of the cancer cells, matches the frequency, then returns it to the cells causing disintegration.
(*Alternative Medicine Digest, issue 20, November 1997*).

+

Although Rife is known to have used audio range frequencies, and experimenters know audio is effective, it should be obvious Rife had to have used frequencies of a range well above audio to cause frequency resonance (illumination) of particles for viewing under his Universal Microscope. According to information from John Crane, Rife used frequencies in the light range of 13 million to 43 million cycles per second to resonate viruses to the point of illumination under the Rife Virus Universal Microscope.

Audio, being a sub-harmonic of higher frequencies, is obtainable with inexpensive equipment as compared to equipment required for the mega- or gigahertz or higher range. For the purpose, audio frequency generators in the range of about 10 hz to 10,000 hz (cycles) are sufficient. Of course, carrier waves are of much higher range.

Research of much higher frequencies, including those in the light wave frequency range may be of future interest — to someone with proper equipment. (Laser?)

Increasing operational power places heavy load demands on components which, in turn, creates excessive heat. One alteration leads to another. A new experimenter should stick to basics until they understand the system before attempting modifications.

One problem that has surfaced many times is the result of electronic engineers with many years of expertise and education who examine the basics of Rife plasma construction with jaundiced eye and immediately 'improve' on the system. As a result, their systems often fail to produce results and they write it off as 'unworkable'! There is an expression that applies:

'there is a method to the madness'. What it amounts to is the expert will insist on 'cleaning up a dirty wave form'. Ironically, it is the dirty wave form that produces results. What modern engineers consider to be a 'dirty wave form' seems in fact, a critical and integral component of true Rife technology and application.

Some basic (experimental) audio frequencies (hertz): 20 - 120 - 440 - 523 - 666 - 728 - 787 - 800 - 880 - 2008 - 2050 - 2080 - 2127 - 4400 - 5K - 10K. (Although 5K & 10K are commonly used experimental frequencies, beginners should use with caution.)

International system of metric units:
kilo	K	10(3rd power)	1,000
mega	M	10(6th power)	1,000,000
giga	G	10(9th power)	1,000,000,000
tera	T	10(12th power)	1,000,000,000,000
peta	P	10(15th power)	1,000,000,000,000,000

Rife's main frequency group:
Bacillus coli—rod form	800 cps
Carcinoma	2128
Gonorrhea	712
Pneumococci	776
Sarcoma	2008
Staphylococci	728
Streptothrix	784
Tetanus	120
Typhoid	1862
Treponema	660
Tuberculosis—rod	803

Chapter Eighteen

Construction Basics:

The following is an intentionally vague overview of basic plasma emission device construction. Before proceeding with any form of construction or experimentation, do read the disclaimers within this publication. (I leave construction techniques to experts!) The author's intent is to only outline the basics. The author is not an electronics oriented person. But, it does prove, if someone with such limited capabilities can construct a working device; then, it is within the means of the average person — with determination. This also indicates why the medical industry is so firmly against frequency healing — imagine ill persons being able to resolve their own illness, including cancerous conditions, on their own terms, without life threatening surgery, chemotherapy and radiation! Unfortunately, it does threaten the health of the illness industry.

Knowledge of CB radio use and setup would be beneficial. Basically, the system would include a method to create and transmit a carrier wave, and a device to generate frequencies which would be transmitted over the carrier wave. Dr. Rife used a phanotron tube as an antenna. The phanotron was directional, meaning the output beam could be directed to a target. And, of course, a power supply of the correct voltage and current requirements. Tubes, less costly than phanotron tubes can be used, especially for experimentation.

A well constructed unit would include an RF shield which, in itself, can be complex. There exists debate regarding the use of audio frequencies; however, documentation does indicate Rife did use audio frequencies — at least to some degree.

Selecting the proper frequency is a difficult issue. To find the correct frequency the best method would be live organisms under a scope while selecting frequencies. We know Rife did perform this very time consuming and tedious task over many long hours. Rife did eventually narrow the selection down to fifteen most useful frequencies.

Another time consuming method is to scan; meaning, on a daily basis, run through a set of frequencies and see what takes place. Use no more than fifteen frequencies at a time. Then, if a reaction occurs the experimenter can backtrack and pinpoint the frequency that caused the reaction. Reactions might be an instant response such as a tingling sensation or a sharp pain in a specific area. Or, a person may not feel anything. When the author's fibromyalgia suddenly disappeared nothing was felt during the scanning process. The total effect was not recognized until the following morning. For the first time in over eight months, the author got out of bed without the usual agonizing pain. It took several minutes to realize a miraculous event had taken place!

To avoid the trials and tribulation of constructing a device, the author recommends purchase of a construction manual. (See resources in rear of book.) Follow links to other resources including component availability and frequency listings. (*Option: do internet search for assembled units.*)

Although researchers of Rife technology have not encountered hazardous effects it must be stated that frequency treatments and experimentation may possibly be dangerous. Let the reader be warned! Review the disclaimer!

Glass (Tubes) and Gases

Tubes and gases are an important and integral part of Rife plasma technology. Initially, Rife used converted X-ray tubes made by Coolidge of General Electric. The tubes were filled with helium gas and up to 8,000 volts applied. Amplification power was 500 watts.

These tubes used a cathode set on an angle of 45 degrees and an anode and a means to apply energy to begin the ionization process These are called phanotron tubes. The phanotron is a diode which restricts current flow to one direction. A directional beam is created. Rife's tube construction included quartz glass.

Due to the type of construction required, phanotron tubes are costly. To keep cost down and to be in a position to experiment with various gases, gas pressure, type of glass and other factors, less sophisticated tubes are used by present day experimenters. These tubes are made using basic techniques as used in neon sign shops using conventional glass tubing. However, requirements for plasma technology is more stringent than conventional neon sign artistry. Thorough evacuation of the tube is critical as slight contamination of the glass or gas will create a number of problems and variable effects.

Noble gases (inert gases), constitute a group of gaseous chemical elements of group 18 of the periodic table. Helium is one of six noble gases. In order of increasing atomic weight they are: helium, neon, argon, krypton, xenon and radon. Note that helium is the lightest of the gases. **Did this factor serve a purpose in Rife's experimentation?**

Argon is commonly used in experimental tubes. Argon is quite effective and provides good results. Neon is another commonly used gas, offering milder effects.

Glass content and gas used in plasma emission devices may affect quality of radiant emission. But, at this point, little is understood as to what effect this may or may not have.

Ions in the gaseous state make up the state of matter known as *plasma*. In the Rife tube, plasma is represented by the glowing gas in the tube. *The Rife tube is an ionization chamber.* Gases may be mixed. For example: 20% neon mixed with 80% argon make tube ignition easier. A small amount of mercury may be used as a starter, as it has been for decades in fluorescent tubes; however, toxic effects of mercury has substantially curbed its use. In addition, experts claim, mercury may produce harmful radiation.

Gas filled tubes operate under negative pressure—vacuum. Millimeters of mercury, torr and pascall are units for measuring the degree of vacuum. Torr, named after Evangelista Torricelli and pascal, after Blaise Pascal. Pascal, being more definitive, is the present day standard in physics. Tube pressure plays a role in tube ignition and generated heat.

For our purpose plasma tubes do not require integrated ignition electrodes but they do serve a purpose in tube construction and maintenance. Tubes may be of various configurations: straight, straight with one or more bubbles, spiral, 'U' shaped.

Glass may be standard silica/lead, Pyrex (trade name), or, quartz. Quartz is preferred by many for various reasons, one of which is favorable transmission of radiation. Quartz and Pyrex are preferred for gases that run hot, such as helium. Quartz may offer unseen characteristics yet undefined!

Basic glass composition is silica, as derived from sand. Commonly used glass is soda-lime as used in bottles, house wares, light bulbs and window glass.

Glass construction includes many variable ingredients to alter composition for specific purposes. Among them are: lead carbonates, phosphates and boron. Neon tubing is standard silica/lead. For heat resistant glass products, as in household wares, borates are added.

Color is a representation of frequency. Therefore, some experimenters place emphasis on plasma color. It seems logical; yet, a tube that provided me with best overall results was 'technically incorrect'. It was a faded white, similar to an 'old' fluorescent tube. Plasma color will vary with type gas, gas pressure, voltage, applied frequency, efficiency of the apparatus and other factors. Plasma color may fade with age and use.

Some experimenters feel the plasma effects and claim certain gases give different effects, such as warm or harsh feeling. Most feel nothing. However, feeling and effectiveness are two different issues. One may not feel anything; yet, achieve results - which is what really counts!

Photons are not fully understood but many experimenters consider photons to play an integral part in overall effect of radiation emission technology. *A photon is a small unit of light energy or electromagnetic radiation. Max Planck and Albert Einstein discovered that light sometimes acts in the manner of a stream of energy particles labeled photons.*

*In laboratory culture testing it seems Rife was able to achieve provable results simply with a brief flashing of the phanotron tube — a duration of just a few seconds.

This all indicates we have a lot of work ahead to sort out variables, define operational standards and design equipment to meet and prove our goals.

Point of Information: Noble gases are available in several grades. Ultra High Purity has less impurities. (This is sometimes referred to as 'lab quality'.) This should be considered an area of importance for radiant plasma technology. It would also be logical to deal with a tube maker who has experience in creating plasma tubes. Anyone who has experimented with plasma technology has likely encountered problems with improperly constructed tubes. There is a difference!

Gas Impurities: Impurities in gas include: oxygen, water, carbon dioxide, nitrogen, carbon monoxide. Although impurities generally create unwanted problems, perhaps some of these impurities could be to our advantage. Of course, that will require diligent and delicate research to determine.

Mercury: Mercury has been used for decades as a starter for gas filled tubes, such as fluorescent. Rifers have used minute amounts of mercury to enhance plasma tube ignition. However, experts claim mercury produces harmful ultra violet rays.

Ions and Plasma: Ions, ionization and plasma are complex issues beyond the scope of this publication. In basic terms, *ions* are formed by addition or removal of electrons from an electrically neutral atomic or molecular configuration. *Plasma (physics):* an electrically neutral, highly ionized gas composed of ions, electrons, and neutral particles. A gas becomes a plasma when the kinetic energy of the gas particles rises to equal the ionization energy of the gas. One method of changing a gas to plasma is introduction of high-energy electrons. *In the Rife tube this may be the result of the RF (radio frequency) component. (Re: Dictionary/MS Encarta.)*

Chapter Nineteen

Back Tracking:

Synopsis of a Press release - dated 1949:

In San Diego, Dr. James Couche, MD, claimed he and other researchers, had confirmed the cancer germ theory held by Dr. Rife, many years prior. Recent studies had been published by two New York research doctors through the Archibald Cancer Research fund at McGill University in Montreal, Canada.

This brought a resurgence in Rife's previous research, studies and theories. Orthodox advocates had denied Rife's claims and refused acceptance. But, recent research revitalized Rife's concepts. When questioned, Rife elaborated on his previous findings of fifteen years prior. Rife explained that he had previously reproduced a fungoid organism and was able to distill the virus back again. **Rife stated he was able to accomplish this cycle 104 times and was able to successfully produce cancer in hundreds of animals with the virus.**

Dr. Couch had returned from a class reunion in Canada which caused the revival of interest in Rife's germ theory. This was the result of Dr. Hett of Windsor, Canada who had developed a cancer serum from a virus which was successful in combating cancer.

Dr. Couch stated that the germ theory explained why surgical treatment of cancer was often unsatisfactory. Dr. Couch favored the germ theory and the serum approach to cancer. The doctor also felt if the germ theory was correct, then cancer could be considered a communicable disease. (Actually, a number of researchers endorsed this theory!)

An advocate of Dr. Hett stated that Hett's work was startling and revolutionary. The supporting doctor had visited Dr. Hett's clinic and, after interviewing 72 patients, found the results amazing. Some of the patients who had recovered from cancer as a result of the serum, had been cancer free up to fourteen years. The supporting doctor strongly recommended that Dr. Hett receive funding for further evaluation of his serum research.

In review of Royal Rife's frequency research and scientific evaluation, here are some basics as taken from documentation.

Rife theorized that the lethal frequencies exist in the organism itself. Therefore, by generating an equivalent frequency, or sympathetic resonance, the organism is set into vibratory mode. If the vibration is strong enough and prolonged enough, the organism will disintegrate. Chemical constituents are known to contain individual frequencies or distinct wave lengths. Since organisms are constituted of various chemicals, the organisms have varying wave lengths. According to Rife, this was confirmed by certain British medical researchers. (**This may have been the British group involved in the 'Beam Ray' entanglement.**)

Viewed under Rife's microscope, the organisms react to specific frequencies. Some organisms literally disintegrate. Others writhe as in agony and gather in unmoving clusters. The correct exposure causes reaction within seconds, according to Rife. After the organisms have been bombarded, laboratory tests show they have become devitalized and no longer exhibit life. They do not propagate their kind and do not produce disease when introduced to test animals.

It was stated that in order to find the correct frequencies, Rife simply kept turning dials and with each turn would study the reaction under the scope. He would do this until he found frequencies that produced the desired results. Strictly trial and error. Later, Rife was assisted by laboratory technician, Henry Siner. As each frequency was recorded, they would start over on the next virus and repeat the procedure. Multitudes of tests were run. They cultivated organisms, searched for frequencies, inoculated the treated organisms into test animals.

Hoyland joined the research group. Per Rife: "Hoyland and Rife built better and better devices for generating and testing frequencies." They eventually recorded frequencies which would produce positive results with repeatability. (However, as we have learned, at a later period of time, failures became prevalent as a result of 'the human factor'.)

'The Daily Californian , August 11, 1971':
'Scientific Genius Dies; Saw work Discredited'

The death of Royal Raymond Rife was announced. Apparently as the result of previously known information it stated: "Rife had lived to see some of his most important work discredited by the medical profession". The article told how (Rife) frequency instruments, used by some doctors across the United States in treating a variety of diseases, were confiscated. It went on to state that reputations of prominent medical researchers and doctors were ruined and one of Rife's associates served three years in prison before winning a reversal of his conviction on grand theft charges." (*Author's note: grand theft referring to money accepted for use of the frequency devices!*)

When John Crane appealed his 1960 conviction he filed an affidavit written by Royal Rife which stated: "Having spent every dime I earned in my research for the benefit of mankind, I have ended up as a pauper, but I achieved the impossible and would do it again."

Rife and the Impossible:

Rife truly was a genius! He had the rare capacity to design and create what was required to accomplish his goals. He did not allow the impossible to stand in his way! *The principle on which the prismatic virus microscope was founded was 'impossible', according to optical engineers! Pleomorphism, as well as isolation and identification of virus forms as accomplished by Rife was 'impossible', according to research experts! Experts had declared many of Rife's achievements as impossible!*

One would assume performing the impossible would lead to fame and accreditation! In reality, it is quite the opposite — the experts who have had their bubbles burst and their egos deflated, take quite a harsh view of 'an outsider' who dispels their combined theories and viewpoints. Instead of acclamation, Rife became the target of ridicule, defamation and destruction. Those who supported Rife were targeted for a similar fate!

Rife Technology — today!

Present day Rife researchers face many obstacles! Some true Rife documentation is held by individuals hoping for financial gain. Some claim 'ownership' of Rife technology, intimidating anyone who attempts to bring the technology in the open. Some claim only their devices are 'true Rife' devices. All of this slows the revival process as well as discrediting a truly remarkable concept!

Chapter Twenty

Mysteries and Oddities:

The Green Ray:

Royal Raymond Rife did the impossible. But, closed minds, dogmatic science, protectionism, won out. Rife and his secrets were buried together. Researchers attempting to retrieve the numerous secrets Rife unveiled have encountered some interesting mysteries. One of these is the case of the 'Green Ray'.

It seems, during research, while experimenting with an X-ray type tube, Rife discovered a greenish/blue ray. Rife apparently considered the ray hazardous since, to protect himself, Rife developed a salt based solution with which he immersed his hands during exposure. After experimenting, he would thoroughly wash his hands.

Super-regeneration:

In a news article, November 3, 1929, Rife made issue of a fact which he considered of great importance — in order to develop the 'super-regenerative ray' he had to work out a method of changing the polarization of vacuum tubes at will — which he did.

Again, in reference to the super-regenerative ray we find these words in a news article: "One revolutionary idea after another followed in the evolution of this apparatus. In its final form the juice runs all around the room, through one gadget or another, and finally feeds through a platinum electrode in a quartz tube filled with helium gas. *These are a few of the refinements that make it 17 times as penetrating as the X-ray."*

Cells - to Infinity-?

In an interview Rife offered very intriguing insight into cell construction. With the tremendous magnification of the Universal Microscope, combined with his expertise, he viewed and photographed evidence that what he termed a 'pinpoint cell', when viewed internally, contains smaller cells and those cells contain even smaller cells. This apparently represented the extent of magnification of his scope since, at that point, he offered conjecture as to where infinity really is! (A very intriguing hypothesis!)

The 'Cure' Word:

Rife urged fellow researchers never to use the 'cure' word. He had witnessed many who had used the 'cure' word in publication and shortly after were attacked and destroyed by the AMA/FDA for making claims of 'cure'! This may be the reason Rife used the word 'devitalize' extensively.

Operation/Location:

Many peculiarities exist in electricity and electronics, in particular in magnetic forces and interaction. Location may be a factor as to where a radiant emission plasma device is placed. Earth wide grid patterns as well as magnetic direction of the device (particularly the emission tube) may play an integral part in effectiveness. Further experimentation may clarify this point. Or, perhaps it is meaningless!

Final Chapter

John Crane

Over the decades since Rife first initiated his concepts, developed equipment and proved efficacy, a constant war has raged over control of Rife technology. Several factions are involved.

*One faction wants control so they can denounce Rife and silence Rife technology for ever.

*Another faction has battled over 'ownership' of Rife technology for control and future profit. **(This is not to be confused with producers of devices or manuals allowing construction of Rife type devices! These people actually help by promoting, distributing and advancing Rife type technology.)**

*Still another group simply wishes to restore Royal Rife (and his concepts) to the world and give Rife long overdue credit for his place in medical history.

Although John Crane's involvement is controversial, we must give him credit for reestablishing Rife's work many years after it had been suppressed. John paid a heavy price. Those who knew him claim prison changed John.

What is more disturbing centers around a bitter battle that took place between John Crane and 'a group' that attempted to take away the Rife Microscope John had in his possession, along with other related equipment and important records. (This was after the death of Rife.)

It seems an investment group was formed which initially included John Crane. The intended purpose was to reverse engineer the Rife Virus Universal Prismatic Microscope to construct, test and market it. Although John Crane signed a corporate contract, John claimed the contract was rewritten at a later date, to exclude and eliminate him from the corporate venture. John then filed a law suit against over twenty defendants involved in what John termed, "a corporate scam and conspiracy of corporations designed to fleece plaintiff which were set up to seize the Rife Universal Microscope."

Prior to the law suit, John had been involved in a serious automobile accident which resulted in head surgery. When John discovered he was being forced out of the corporation he attempted to retrieve the microscope. During the attempted retrieval process, John claimed, "defendant (xxxx) pummeled plaintiff on the head knowing of his brain operation with the intent of murder".

John was about 73 years old at this time, had spent time in prison, with little finances left and little to show for his involvement in his attempted revival of Rife technology. His bitterness toward the entire affair by this time can be well imagined.

Possibly in an attempt to save money, John handled some of the litigation processing himself which proved disastrous since improper procedures created loopholes for the defendants and weakened John's position. It seems, the case was not resolved. John died a few years later.

John Crane remains an enigmatic, controversial character. Depending on definition, he was sincere, reliable and dedicated. On the other side, he was stubborn, offensive and abrasive. He seems to have made more enemies than friends. But, the fact remains, John did much to preserve Rife history and technology!

Strange Event:

In an attempt to avoid controversy or discredit of this material, *conspiratorial issues* have been side stepped. However, there is one issue that must be commented on — *chem-trails*! For those unfamiliar with this phenomenon, an internet search is suggested. For those familiar, the following will be self explanatory!

This is in reference to *Chapter Ten, Case History*, regarding the statement whereas a sudden change in health condition required a catheter followed by radical prostatectomy; triggered by yet to be explained circumstances! *Here is a clue to that event*!

My health problems were under control until a *strange event* took place! My employment required working all over the local county. As a result I spent two days in an area near a military air base. During that period the sky above was a checker board of chem-trails, crisscrossing from horizon–to–horizon, completely covering the sky. I had heard of this phenomenon but until then had not considered it a reality. It was something extraordinary, unnatural, even sinister!

Three days later I came down with a 'flu like condition'. Two weeks after that a catheter was required, followed by surgery a few weeks later! The surgeon had no explanation for my sudden change and after surgery he commented that what he encountered was unusual, but he did not elaborate!

Let the reader decide!

Update:

As this book is being written, new information is being uncovered regarding the life of Rife along with new developments in application of Rife technology.

Workable frequencies are being discovered and made available through diligent research making it easier for new researchers to join in and probe the merits of frequency healing.

Construction of such devices has become easier with specially developed components making the entire process and application more rewarding. For example, a frequency generator and pulser (previously separate components), can now be obtained in a single, compact, programmable unit, which not only performs the above but offers additional features of regulating duration (length of time), duty cycle, and many other options. For computer buffs, programs are available enabling researchers to computerize Rife technology.

Rife technology may have finally reached the point where it cannot be stopped by medical monopoly. The unfortunate aspect may be abuse by fast buck entrepreneurs. It is imperative that researchers know who they are dealing with and what they are getting for their money. Implication of true Rife plasma emission technology is often confusing and misleading. Some manufacturers command outrageous prices for electronic gadgets containing a few dollars worth of electronic parts passing them off as 'Rife' devices. This is not to say these devices don't work — they can work well for certain applications if properly engineered and produced by competent technicians. But, do they represent true Rife plasma emission technology? For that matter many die hard Rifers question whether any technology presently available can be construed as true Rife technology. But, if it works, does that matter?

Conclusion

The purpose of this publication is to encourage public interest in the merits of Rife technology and the suppression of a possible solution to the ills of humanity. Only through expanded, individual research can one truly make a justifiable analysis. What is done with the material, research and the final conclusion might well play an important roll in the future of our health needs.

It is doubtful the impenetrable wall of protectionism constructed by the medical industry will ever be breached. For that matter, possibly they are justified in their goals. But, that is for someone else to decide. One thing is certain, the cost of medical care is outstripping the economy of the nation 'and our assets'.

In any event, choice of health treatment should be an individual decision. The law should not be used to force individuals into unwanted health care and the law should not be used to prevent treatment of choice.

Medical lobbyists are big spenders with unlimited financial resources. How can the public expect protection from our representatives when those representatives have effectively been 'neutralized' by campaign funds, various forms of financial assistance and stock holdings?

The advancement of electromedicine has clearly been suppressed for eighty years in the United States due to greed and power of the existing medical system. In other countries where medical advancement has not been held back, electromedicine has made great strides. Present day European medical researchers have combined Rife's work with modern electronics creating solid state, compact yet powerful devices that offer amazing healing capabilities. Medical practitioners, in some countries combine modern technology with the wisdom of the ancients. The United States may have lost a great science!

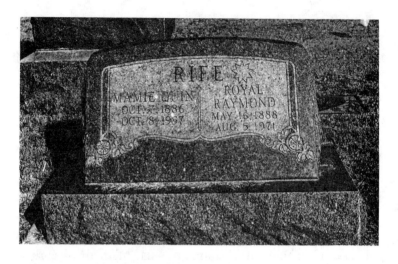

Photo By Gerald Foye (Author).

Headstone located in Mount Hope Cemetery, San Diego, California:

"Rife, Mamie Quin, Oct 7, 1886—Oct 8, 1957
Rife, Royal Raymond, May 16, 1888—August 5, 1971"

Does the secret to the Rife Ray lie buried here?

The Last Word: (Philosophical Perspective!)

On the other side of the coin, each successive generation seems more bent toward self destruction with consumption of illicit drugs, rampant crime and corresponding violence. One might wonder if there is higher authority than the medical monopoly behind our failure for a simpler solution to our health problems. Perhaps we really are not ready for Rife technology; but, for reasons we cannot comprehend!

Serious Experimenters:
　　For the reader who may be seriously considering experimenting with Rife frequency technology, first, review the *disclaimer* at the front of this book. The next step is to start off in the proper direction. On that basis it is recommended to consider purchase of a frequency emission plasma device construction manual as authored by James Bare. The manual offers easy to follow instructions utilizing readily available components and sources for components. Assembling the system yourself allows the builder many options: ability to understand the system making it relatively easy to troubleshoot, experiment with different components, adjust to any frequency 'within the range of the equipment' and many other options.

Title: Resonant Frequency Therapy, Building The Rife Beam Ray Device.
Contact:
James E. Bare D.C.
8005 Marble Ave. NE
Albuquerque, NM 87110 USA

Phone: (voice) 505-268-4272, (Fax): 505-254-7884

rifetech@rt66.com
http://www.rt66.com/~rifetech/

　　For experimenters with no aptitude for self construction, completed Bare Rife units may be available. Contact James Bare or follow *internet links*.

(James Bare must be given credit for his roll in revival and sharing of Rife technology on layman terms.)

Beam Ray

Lynn Kenny, head of present day Beam Ray, has been instrumental in pending research of medical application of Rife related technology. Beam Ray company manufactures plasma devices for research programs.

(The name Beam Ray is not to be confused with the Beam Ray Corporation and related court trials of 1938/1939.)

Beam Ray
9220-A1 Parkway East
Birmingham, AL 35206

(205) 841-6554

*There are many producers of Rife related and so-called, Rife related devices. Some are excellent, backed up with sincere and honest research efforts. However, an interested Rife enthusiast should use caution. Serious 'homework' is in order before making a decision and selection!

Unfortunately, due to legal requirements, claims to cure are not allowable according to existing FDA regulations. This creates difficulties for genuine research efforts and adds to the confusion of researching a device; or, for that matter, any medical alternative!

A word on resources and other information relating to the advancement of Rife technology: Until a person has actually faced trials and tribulations surrounding major health problems; and, until a person has actually faced persecution while attempting to gain access to personal choices to resolve health issues, it is impossible to truly comprehend the barriers, restrictions, and misinformation a medical victim must face.

Many persons have discovered there is no limit or expense certain forces will go to in order to control what they perceive to be their rightful rulership over the health industry.

Therefore, when sorting information available in libraries, internet; or, other sources, be wary of intentional misinformation.

There are well funded organizations designed to mislead and discredit alternative medical applications. Some websites are set up in such a manner as to appear to be in favor of alternatives; then, guide the unwary searcher off to sites designed to discredit the alternative the individual is examining.

Many websites have been forced to shut down. Websites are constantly changing location and address. Therefore, the following websites may not be available or have relocated which will require further search.

RESOURCES:
Subject to change.

Suggested sources for further research:
Books:
The Healing Of Cancer, by Barry Lynes ISBN 0-919951-44-9
The Body Electric, by Robert O. Becker, MD & Gary Selden, ISBN 0-688-06971-1
Rife Way 111, by Mark A. Simpson
Tesla - Man Out Of Time, Margaret Cheney. ISBN 0-440-39077-x
Racketeering In Medicine By James Carter ISBN 1-878901-32-x
The Social Transformation of American Medicine. ISBN 0465079342
Consumer guides are available to cover prescription drug side effects.

Rife device construction manual: 'Resonant Frequency Therapy - Building The Rife Beam Ray Device', By James E. Bare: http://www.rt66.com/~rifetech/

Don Tunney: **http://www.Kalamark.com/devices/**
http://www.rifetechnology.com
Other experimental plasma device:
http://www.flinet.com/~vibrnthealth
http://web.idirect.com/~showcase/althealth/index.htm
http://www.rifeworks.com

Rife site with most complete historical, technical information and major links: **http://rife.org/index.htm**

Rife type device: Bio-Ray, Beam Ray LLC., 9220 A-1 Parkway East, Birmingham, AL 35206. 205-841-6554

Frequency lists
Many frequency lists are available - follow links from Rife home pages for up to date listings.

Resources (continued):

Recommended sites or :keywords:
Ralph Moss (Book author): http://www.ralphmoss.com/index.html
Tesla
Lakhovsky-Multiple Wave Oscillator
Royal Rife
Morris Fishbein
AMA, FDA
William F. Koch: http://williamfkoch.com/texts/martyr/Martyr.htm
Max Gerson - Gerson Clinic
Stanislaw Burzynski

Harry Hoxsey - Hoxsey Clinic: Excellent study of Hoxsey and other alternative treatments by Patricia Spain Ward PhD (1988), http://members.tripod.com/hoxsey/ward.html
Hoxsey video - Excellent documentary on alternative medical suppression: "How Healing Becomes A Crime": ISBN 1-885538-76-6
www.wellmedia.com   email:mail@wellmedia.com

REPORTS (To review):
The Fitzgerald Report (Medical politics):

For detailed information of the Rife Virus Universal Microscope:
Journal Of The Franklin Institute, Feb 1944. The New Microscopes, By R.E. Seidel, MD and M. Elizabeth Winter. Re: Rife's scope.
Smithsonian Institution: The Universal Microscope, from the Annual Report of the Board of Regents of The Smithsonian Institution - 1944.